Clinics in Human Lactation

Non-Pharmacological Treatments for Depression in New Mothers

Evidence-based Support of Omega-3s, Bright Light Therapy, Exercise, Social Support, Psychotherapy, and St. John's Wort

Kathleen Kendall-Tackett, Ph.D., IBCLC

Clinics in Human Lactation

Non-Pharmacological Treatments for Depression in New Mothers

Evidence-based Support of Omega-3s, Bright Light Therapy, Exercise, Social Support, Psychotherapy, and St. John's Wort

Kathleen Kendall-Tackett, Ph.D., IBCLC
University of New Hampshire

Praeclarus Press, LLC
2504 Sweetgum Lane
Amarillo, Texas 79124 USA
806-367-9950
www.PraeclarusPress.com

DISCLAIMER

The information contained in this publication is advisory only and is not intended to replace sound clinical judgment or individualized patient care. The author disclaims all warranties, whether expressed or implied, including any warranty as the quality, accuracy, safety, or suitability of this information for any particular purpose.

ISBN: 9781939807984

TABLE OF CONTENTS

Non-Pharmacological Treatments for Depression in New Mothers

Evidence-based Support of Omega-3s, Bright Light Therapy, Exercise, Social Support, Psychotherapy, and St. John's Wort

For many women, the lovely images of life with a new baby are a lie. Instead of feeling happy, they feel overwhelmed with their new role—and anything but blissful. In a recent survey of 1,573 American new mothers, nearly two out of three had depressive symptoms in the previous two weeks (Lowe, 2007). Approximately 10% to 20% of mothers will develop postpartum depression. In high-risk populations, that percentage can be as high as 40% to 50% (Kendall-Tackett, 2005).

If mothers are depressed, helping them weigh their treatment options is one specific way to assist them. While not recommending specific treatments, information can be given to them about which treatments work and how they impact breastfeeding. This monograph summarizes current research on non-pharmacologic treatments for depression and describes specific steps mothers can take. Many of these modalities can be used alone, as adjuncts to antidepressants, or in combination with each other. All are compatible with breastfeeding. But first, it's important to understand why depression needs to be addressed in the first place.

CONSEQUENCES OF UNTREATED POSTPARTUM DEPRESSION

The consequences of postpartum depression are simply too serious to ignore. We can't just hope that it will resolve or go away on its own. This section briefly reviews the literature on depression's harmful effects for both mother and baby.

Consequences for Mothers

Depression is quite damaging to women's health. For a number of years, researchers have known that depression compromises the immune system by decreasing lymphocyte count and natural killer cell cytotoxicity (Robles *et al.*, 2005; Weisse, 1992). This increases women's vulnerability to infection, a finding that Groër and colleagues (Groër *et al.*, 2005b) recently confirmed. When mothers in their study were stressed or depressed, both mother and baby had increased rates of infection.

More recently, researchers have discovered that depression increases the risk of chronic diseases, such as heart disease, metabolic syndrome, and diabetes (Robles *et al.*, 2005). Depression is associated with other serious health problems, including chronic pain, impaired wound healing, and even Alzheimer's disease (Kiecolt-Glaser *et al.*, 2005; Wilson *et al.*, 2002). Discussing the connection between depression and heart disease, Kop and Gottdiener (2005) hypothesized that depression in early adulthood promotes vascular injury and may encourage lipid and macrophage deposits. For people with preexisting cardiovascular disease, depression-induced chronic inflammation reduces the stability of plaque which can lead to acute cardiac episodes. And while cardiovascular events are less likely in a population of new mothers, these studies illustrate depression's serious health effects.

Unfortunately, even mild-to-moderate depression has a negative impact. In one study, Weinberg and colleagues (2001) compared women with subclinical depression to both non-depressed women and women with postpartum major depression. Women with subclinical depression had poorer psychosocial functioning than non-depressed women and were comparable to those with major depression. They also had more negative and less positive affect with their babies, lower self-esteem, and were less confident as mothers.

Depression can also impair women's relationships. Depressed women report more communication problems with their partners and have marital dysfunction that persists long after the depression has resolved (Roux *et al.*, 2002). In a study that compared women who were currently depressed to those with a history of depression and to those with no history of depression, the depressed and formerly depressed women were impaired on every measure of interpersonal behavior, had less stable marriages, and reported lower levels of marital satisfaction than women with no history of depression (Hammen & Brennan, 2002).

Consequences of Maternal Depression for Babies

Depression is also potentially quite harmful for babies, as numerous studies have demonstrated, with children ranging in age from infancy to young adulthood. Children of depressed mothers have more social, behavioral, and cognitive difficulties than their counterparts with non-depressed mothers.

A study of 48 neonates found that babies of depressed mothers had abnormal electroencephalogram (EEG) activation patterns and elevated cortisol levels (Field *et al.*, 2002). They also had more state-change variability during sleep/wake observations and had impaired performance on the Neonatal Behavior Assessment Scale. In an American sample of 5,000 mother-infant pairs, children of depressed mothers had more behavior problems and lower vocabulary scores at age five (Brennan *et al.*, 2000). When mothers' depression was severe and chronic, the children had more behavior problems. The same was true if mothers had had more recent episodes of depression.

Researchers from Finland examined the long-term effects of postpartum depression on children's social competence (Luoma *et al.*, 2001). Children whose mothers had postpartum depression or whose mothers were currently depressed had lower social competence at ages 8 to 9. Social competence included parents' reports of children's activities, hobbies, tasks, and chores; functioning in social relationships; and school achievements. Mothers were assessed for depression during pregnancy, immediately postpartum, and when their children were eight to nine years old.

The impact of parental depression can even last into adulthood. A 20-year follow-up of children of depressed mothers and fathers compared them with a matched group of children whose parents had no psychiatric illness. The adult children of depressed parents had three times the rate of major depression, anxiety disorders, and substance abuse compared with children of non-depressed parents. In addition, children of depressed parents had higher rates of medical problems and premature mortality (Weissman *et al.*, 2006).

Fortunately, the news is not all bad. The Jones and colleagues' (2004) study provides an exception to the bleak picture of the effects of maternal depression on babies. This study compared four groups of postpartum women: depressed women who were either breast- or bottle-feeding and non-depressed women who were either breast- or bottle-feeding. The outcome was illustrated by babies' electroencephalogram (EEG) patterns. In studies of maternal depression, babies of depressed mothers frequently have abnormal EEG patterns. These abnormal patterns are similar to patterns seen in chronically depressed adults. Babies of depressed, breastfeeding mothers had normal EEG patterns. In contrast, babies of depressed, non-breastfeeding women did not. In other words, breastfeeding protected babies from the harmful effects of maternal depression. The authors observed that depressed, breastfeeding mothers touched, stroked, and made eye contact with their babies more than depressed, non-breastfeeding women because these behaviors are built into the breastfeeding relationship. This is one more reason to encourage and support breastfeeding in depressed mothers. These findings also encourage us to offer specific guidance to depressed, non-breastfeeding mothers so they continue to interact with their babies while they recover from depression.

THE CHALLENGE OF PERINATAL DEPRESSION: RISK/BENEFIT ANALYSES OF PHARMACOLOGIC VERSUS NON-PHARMACOLOGIC TREATMENTS

Because of postpartum depression's devastating effects on both mother and baby, it needs to be identified and treated promptly. Frontline treatments for postpartum depression include antidepressants and psychotherapy. But medications, in particular, present challenges when used in pregnant and breastfeeding women, as Yonkers (2007) describes.

In medicine, there are often situations that require patients and their providers to make difficult management decisions... The treatment of women with depression who are either pregnant or breastfeeding presents a number of issues for which we have insufficient data. These include questions such as: ... What are the short- and long-term consequences for children exposed to maternal psychiatric illness or the long-term consequences for a neonate exposed to an antidepressant as a result of breastfeeding? The absence of sufficient data is not the result of a lack of interest among researchers but derives largely from the ethical or practical issues that make research in this area difficult (p. 1459).

One challenge associated with medicating pregnant and breastfeeding women is making an accurate risk/benefit analysis (Freeman, 2007). Do the risks of the medication outweigh the risks of allowing depression to continue during pregnancy and the puerperium? In most cases, the answer is likely to be yes. But it simply isn't prudent to be glib about this decision since there are some risks associated with using medication—especially during pregnancy. A recent review on safety and effectiveness of antidepressants raised similar concerns. Cipriani and colleagues (2007) noted that antidepressant use in the first trimester may lead to birth defects—although they hastened to add that there is no robust evidence that common antidepressants, such as the SSRIs, cause teratogenic effects.

Similarly, the results of the Sloane Epidemiology Center Birth Defects Study recently confirmed that SSRIs do not significantly increase the risk of birth defects overall. They included three birth defects in their study: craniosynostosis, omphalocele, and heart defects (Louik *et al.*, 2007). However, sertraline increased the risk of omphalocele (odds ratio, 5.7) and septal defects (odds ratio, 2.0), and paroxetine increased the risk of the heart defect right ventricular outflow tract obstruction (odds ratio, 3.3). It should be noted that even with these odds ratios, only 1.7% to 4.7% of infants with these defects were exposed to SSRIs in the first trimester. The authors concluded that the overall risk of having a child affected by SSRI use was only 0.2%.

There are also concerns about using medications during the third trimester. Neonates whose mothers used antidepressants during pregnancy had increased rates of respiratory distress, feeding difficulties, and low birth weight due, in part, to neonatal withdrawal (Cipriani *et al.*, 2007; Looper, 2007; Louik *et al.*, 2007). However, we must weigh the risk of neonatal complications against the risk associated with stopping medications during pregnancy. Women who discontinue their antidepressants during pregnancy are more than twice as likely to relapse compared with women who continue (Looper, 2007). Generally speaking, these medications appear safe when used in the recommended dosages. But the results are mixed and researchers have been expressing concern (Dietz *et al.*, 2007).

With regard to breastfeeding, some have argued that we don't know the clinical significance of medications transferred via breastmilk (Cipriani *et al.*, 2007), nor do we know the long-term effects (Payne, 2007). Commonly cited adverse effects include infant irritability, poor-quality or uneasy sleep, and poor feeding. But most of these effects have been documented in case studies, not larger randomized trials. In contrast, studies with larger samples generally find no adverse effects. Any risk/benefit analysis must also weigh the risks of infant exposure to mother's medications with the risks of not breastfeeding, which can be considerable. In most cases, the risks associated with breastfeeding on medication are still less than the risk of not breastfeeding. There are risks associated with ongoing, untreated maternal depression (Hale, 2006; Payne, 2007).

Considering Depression Severity and Patient Compliance in Treatment Decisions

Depression severity figures into the balance between antidepressant use and risks associated with their use. When a mother's depression is severe, the benefits most likely outweigh the risks (Geddes *et al.*, 2007). The risk/benefit analysis is less clear among patients with milder depression. Does the benefit outweigh the risk in these patients? Should medications remain the frontline treatment for women with mild-to-moderate symptoms? Freeman (2007) suggested that non-pharmacologic choices may be most appropriate for women with mild depression. However, if depression is moderate to severe or if a mother has a history of depression, medications may still be the best first choice.

Patient compliance is another variable to consider. Some mothers will not use medications while breastfeeding—even when assured that their babies are exposed to only a small amount of their dose (Freeman, 2007). Depressed mothers may avoid medications because they worry about how it will affect their babies, that they will become addicted, or because they believe that depression will resolve on its own (Letourneau *et al.*, 2007). With education, some of these mothers may be persuaded to take medications. Indeed, medications may be the best choice for them. But concerns about taking medications while breastfeeding may keep others from seeking treatment altogether (Hendrick, 2003), which brings us to the subject of non-pharmacologic treatments.

Advantages of Non-Pharmacologic Approaches

Non-pharmacologic treatments are widely used in the general population and among patients with psychiatric disorders. In a recent review, Werneke and colleagues (2006) noted that up to 57% of psychiatric patients have used alternative treatments, usually to treat depression and anxiety. From the patient's perspective, non-pharmacologic approaches offer a number of advantages. If you understand why women might prefer these modalities, you can talk more comfortably with them about their choices. Women are more likely to be forthcoming about using them.

☒ **Control:** One reason patients prefer non-pharmacologic treatments is that they can control their own health care. Instead of having to wait for a doctor's appointment, they can address their depression right away. They have control over when they start treatment and when they stop.

☒ **Privacy:** Patients may be ashamed to admit that they are depressed and are frightened by the possibility that their employers or others will find out that they are taking antidepressants. Unfortunately, on occasion, medication information does get released to employers via insurance forms or just plain gossip—even with confidentiality regulations in place. Antidepressant use can influence hiring and promotion decisions in some types of jobs. Even if that's not the case, patients may still not want others to know.

☒ **Costs:** Newer and name-brand antidepressants can be expensive, especially if not covered by insurance. In contrast, non-pharmacologic treatments are generally reasonably priced and can be purchased at discount and warehouse stores. The savings each month can be substantial compared with name-brand, non-generic prescription drugs. This is becoming less of an issue as many popular antidepressants are available in generic form, but it still can be a concern for some mothers.

☒ **Side Effects and Safety:** The side-effect and safety profiles of non-pharmacologic treatments are significantly better than those associated with medications (Klier *et al.*, 2006; Schultz, 2006). For example, the tricyclic antidepressants have anti-cholinergic side effects, including dry mouth, constipation, and blurred vision. The selective serotonin reuptake inhibitors (SSRIs) have sexual side effects, such as inorgasmia. For some, side effects prove intolerable and are a common reason why patients stop taking their medications. Most non-pharmacologic treatments have very low incidence of adverse effects. For example, according to one recent review, risk of adverse events associated with St. John's wort was 10 times lower than with standard antidepressants (Schultz, 2006).

☒ **Patient Compliance:** Patient compliance is an important issue. Just because women are prescribed antidepressants does not mean they will take them. In one recent study of depressed men and women in New York City (N=829), only 28% were still taking their antidepressants three months later (Olfson *et al.*, 2006). Patients were more likely to stop taking them if they were Hispanic, had less than 12 years of education, or were low income. They were more likely to continue taking their medications if they had more than 12 years of education, had participated in psychotherapy at some point, and had private health insurance.

The discussion above highlights why women might choose alternative treatment approaches for postpartum depression. The next section describes some current research on the causes of depression. This research provides a unifying construct that explains why such a wide variety of treatments are all effective. It has to do with the immune system's role in depression.

INFLAMMATION AND DEPRESSION

Researchers have found that systemic inflammation plays a key role in the etiology of depression. When describing this relationship a decade ago, Maes (1998) noted that there are a number of plausible explanations for why inflammation might increase the risk for depression. First, when inflammation levels are high, people experience classic symptoms of depression, such as fatigue, lethargy, and social withdrawal. Researchers discovered this connection when using inflammatory cytokines as treatments for conditions such as cancer or hepatitis. When treated with cytokines, depression increases in a predictable and dose-responsive way: the greater the dose of cytokines, the more depressed the patients (Konsman *et al.*, 2002). Second, inflammation activates the hypothalamic-pituitary-adrenal (HPA) axis, dysregulating levels of cortisol. Cortisol is designed to keep inflammation in check. However, depression dysregulates cortisol's control of the immune response, whereby it no longer restrains the inflammatory response (Dhabhar & McEwen, 2001). Finally, inflammation decreases serotonin by lowering levels of its precursor, tryptophan.

To understand the role of inflammation in depression, it's helpful to first review the stress response—the normal physiologic response to a perceived threat. Inflammation is due to activity of the immune system which is part of

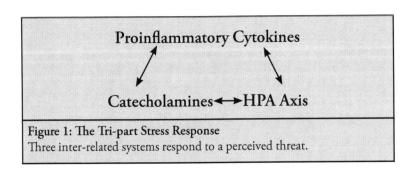

Figure 1: The Tri-part Stress Response
Three inter-related systems respond to a perceived threat.

the three-part stress response.

How Humans Respond to a Perceived Threat

When faced with a threat, human bodies have a number of interdependent mechanisms designed to preserve homeostasis and our lives. This physiologic response is the same for both physical and psychological threats.

The sympathetic nervous system responds first by releasing catecholamines (norepinephrine, epinephrine, and dopamine). This is the fight-or-flight response, and it occurs instantly.

Catecholamines
- Norepinephrine
- Epinephrine
- Dopamine

Figure 2: Catecholamine (Fight-or-Flight Response) Response Neurotransmitters released in response to a perceived threat.

The hypothalamic-pituitary-adrenal (HPA) axis also responds to threat with a cascade of stress hormones. The hypothalamus releases corticotrophin releasing hormone (CRH), which causes the pituitary to release adrenocorticotropin hormone (ACTH), which causes the adrenal cortex to release cortisol, a glucocorticoid.

HPA Axis
- Hypothalamus
- CRH (CRF)
- Pituitary
- ACTH
- Adrenal cortex
- Cortisol

Figure 3: Hypothalamic-Pituitary-Adrenal (HPA) Axis
The cascade of stress hormones released from the three structures of the HPA Axis.

The immune system also responds by increasing inflammation by releasing proinflammatory cytokines. These cytokines cause inflammation and are designed to fight infection and aid in wound healing. But when levels are too

> **Proinflammatory Cytokines**
> - IL-1β   • TNF-α
> - IL-6   • IFN-γ
>
> **Figure 4: Immune Response: Proinflammatory Cytokines**
> The immune system responds to stress by releasing proinflammatory molecules.

high, they increase the risk of depression (Maes, 2001; Robles *et al.*, 2005).

The three systems illustrated in Figure 1 are interrelated, with a series of checks and balance—when the system is working normally. Inflammation influences levels of serotonin and catecholamines and impacts the HPA axis, which controls cortisol. Once inflammation starts, it triggers the HPA axis to release cortisol to keep it under control. McEwen (2003) noted that the stress response has an important role in allostasis—or maintaining homeostasis through change. However, the stress response is meant to be acute, not chronic. When it is "on" when not needed, it can create wear on the system— or allostatic load. Indeed, a chronically activated stress response can damage tissues and organs.

Depression is such a case where the normal checks and balances fail. Cortisol is anti-inflammatory and is generally secreted when inflammation levels get too high. However, depressed people either have abnormally low levels of cortisol, or they become less sensitive to it. In either case, cortisol does not restrain the inflammatory response. Groër and Morgan (2007), in their study of 200 postpartum women, noted a downregulation of the HPA axis and abnormally low levels of cortisol in depressed women at 4 to 6 weeks postpartum.

Another study of 72 women had similar findings (Miller *et al.*, 2005). Depressed and non-depressed women were exposed to a stressor in the form of a mock job interview. Researchers then drew blood to assess levels of inflammatory cytokines. They found that stress increased monocytes, neutrophils, C-reactive protein, and proinflammatory cytokines (IL-6 and TNF-α) for all the women in the study. However, the depressed women had a blunted cortisol response to stress and increased resistance to the molecules that normally terminate the inflammatory response. The researchers hypothesized that depression created a long-term decrease in sensitivity to cortisol which allowed inflammation to continue unchecked. These same researchers had similar findings in a sample of parents caring for children with cancer (Miller *et al.*, 2002). This study compared parents of healthy children with parents of ill children. They found that parents of ill children had a blunted response to cortisol and that it didn't restrain inflammation.

Researchers generally assess inflammation by measuring serum levels of proinflammatory cytokines, the messenger molecules of the immune system. These molecules are released by the white blood cells, and they orchestrate the inflammatory response (Miller *et al.*, 2002). The proinflammatory cytokines identified most often in depression research are interleukin-1β(IL-1β), interleukin-6 (IL-6), and tumor necrosis factor-α (TNF-α). Researchers sometimes include other measures of inflammation in their studies. These include interferon-γ (IFN-γ), intercellular adhesion molecule (ICAM), fibrinogen, and C-reactive protein (CRP). Maes (2001) described the stress-depression-inflammation connection as follows:

The discovery that psychological stress can induce the production of proinflammatory cytokines has important implications for human psychopathology and, in particular, for the aetiology of major depression. Psychological stressors, such as negative life events, are emphasized in the aetiology of depression. Thus, psychosocial and environmental stressors play a role as direct precipitants of major depression, or they function as vulnerability factors which predispose humans to develop major depression. Major depression is accompanied by activation of the inflammatory response system (IRS) with, among other things, an increased production of proinflammatory cytokines, such as IL-1β, IL-6, TNF-α, and IFN-γ, signs of monocytic- and T-cell activation, and an acute-phase response (Maes, 2001, p. 193).

In other words, our bodies "translate" physical and psychological stress into inflammation, and it underlies all the other risk factors for depression. Inflammation is not simply a risk factor; it is the risk factor for depression, the one that ties the others together (Kendall-Tackett, 2007a).

Why Inflammation is Particularly Relevant to Depression in New Mothers

Pregnant and postpartum women are particularly vulnerable to this effect because their inflammation levels normally rise during the last trimester of pregnancy—a time when they are also at highest risk for depression (Kendall-Tackett, 2005; 2007a). Indeed, the pattern of elevated cytokine levels in the last trimester matches the pattern of perinatal depression much more accurately than the pattern of other biological markers, such as the rise and fall of reproductive hormones. The findings on women's increased risk of depression during pregnancy versus postpartum are summarized below.

Depression Risk Is Highest During the Last Trimester of Pregnancy

Several studies of perinatal depression have found that a higher percentage of women were depressed during pregnancy than postpartum. In a large study of pregnant women (N=9,028), depression was measured at 18 and 32 weeks gestation and again at eight weeks and eight months postpartum (Evans et al., 2001). The authors found that depression rates were highest at 32 weeks gestation and lowest at eight months postpartum. Similarly, Hobfoll and colleagues (Hobfoll et al., 1995; Ritter et al., 2000) found the highest percentage of depressed women was during pregnancy (28% and 25%), not postpartum (23%). Their sample was 192 low-income women from the inner city. Fifty-three percent of the women with postpartum depression were also depressed during pregnancy.

Twenty-three percent of mothers from India had postpartum depression (N=252). Seventy-eight percent were also depressed during pregnancy, and only 21% developed depression for the first time at six weeks postpartum. Moreover, 59% of women depressed at six weeks were still depressed at six months postpartum (Patel et al., 2002).

In a sample of 80 women, 25% experienced depression during pregnancy, and 16% experienced depression at four-to-five weeks postpartum (Da Costa et al., 2000). Women who were depressed postpartum reported more emotional coping and higher state and trait anxiety during pregnancy. Depressed mood during pregnancy best predicted postpartum depressed mood. In a low-income, ethnic minority sample (N=802), 37% of the women had depressive symptoms, and 6.5% to 8.5% had major depression at three-to-five weeks postpartum. Fifty percent of these women were also depressed during pregnancy (Yonkers et al., 2001).

In a meta-analysis of 84 studies, Beck (2001) found that prenatal depression, prenatal anxiety, and a history of previous depression were all risk factors for postpartum depression, with moderate effect sizes ranging from 0.38 to 0.46. Similarly, O'Hara and Swain's (1996) meta-analysis found that depression and anxiety during pregnancy and a mother's history of psychopathology were moderate-to-strong predictors of postpartum depression.

Not all studies have found increased depression during pregnancy, however. Among 4,398 women whose pregnancies ended in live births, 15% were identified as being depressed either before, during, or after their pregnancies (Dietz *et al.*, 2007). This sample was drawn from a large Health Maintenance Organization in Oregon and Washington State. Nine percent had depression diagnosed before their pregnancies, 6.9% during their pregnancies, and 10.4% after their pregnancies. Of the women who were depressed before pregnancy, 56.4% were also depressed during their pregnancies. Among women depressed postpartum, 54% were also identified as depressed before or during their pregnancies. Seventy-five percent of the depressed women were prescribed an antidepressant. The authors noted that one limitation to their data was that depression was not directly assessed. Only women whom health care providers identified as depressed were included in the depressed group. This methodological issue likely under-represented the true incidence of depression in this population and may have limited the findings.

Depression, Inflammation, and Preterm Birth

Depression poses another health risk to puerperal women—increased risk of preterm birth. Inflammation may explain why (Dayan *et al.*, 2006). Generally speaking, elevated cytokines are adaptive because they help prevent infection. In pregnant women, inflammation also helps prepare their bodies for labor (Coussons-Read *et al.*, 2005). Unfortunately, stressors common to new mothers, such as sleep disturbance, pain, and psychological trauma, also increase inflammation and appear to boost it beyond normal levels (Kendall-Tackett, 2007a).

In a study of 200 women at 4 to 6 weeks postpartum, depressed mothers had significantly smaller babies, more life stress, and more negative life events than mothers who were not depressed (Groër & Morgan, 2007). These women also had abnormally low cortisol levels, meaning that inflammation was not restrained. In a prospective cohort study of 681 women from France, the rate of spontaneous preterm birth for depressed women was more than double that of non-depressed women (9.7% versus 4%; odds ratio=3.3; Dayan *et al.*, 2006). A study in Goa, India (N=270) found that babies of mothers who were depressed during their third trimester were significantly more likely to have low birth weight babies than their non-depressed counterparts. The most depressed mothers were at highest risk (odds ratio, 2.5). This was true even after controlling for other factors that influence birth weight, such as maternal age, maternal and paternal education, and paternal income (Patel & Prince, 2006).

A study of 1,820 women from Baltimore found that women with high levels of anxiety about their pregnancies were significantly more likely to have their babies prematurely (Orr *et al.*, 2007). Indeed, women with the highest levels of pregnancy-related anxiety had three times the risk of preterm birth compared to women with low anxiety. These findings were true even after controlling for traditional risk factors for preterm birth, including first- or second-trimester bleeding, drug use, unemployment, previous preterm or still birth, smoking, low body mass index, maternal education, age, and race.

Dayan and colleagues (2006) speculated on two possible pathways by which depression might lead to preterm birth. First, depression can lead to elevated cortisol levels which increases corticotrophin releasing hormone (CRH). CRH triggers parturition. Second, depression activates the proinflammatory cytokines and prostaglandin E2, which is secreted in response to cortisol and proinflammatory cytokines. Prostaglandin E2 plays a major role in uterine contractions (Dayan *et al.*, 2006).

IL-6 and TNF-α are other possible mechanisms. One function of IL-6 and TNF–α is to ripen the cervix before delivery. In a study of 30 pregnant women, Coussons-Read and colleagues (2005) found that TNF-α and IL-6 levels were significantly higher and the anti-inflammatory cytokine IL-10 was significantly lower in mothers who were stressed compared with mothers who were not stressed. The authors hypothesized that inflammation was the likely mechanism to explain the relationship between maternal stress and preterm birth. They noted that high levels of inflammation (particularly IL-6 and TNF-α) were associated with preeclampsia and premature labor. Infection also increases the risk of preterm delivery, and TNF-α is released in response to both viral and bacterial infections. They concluded that high levels of proinflammatory cytokines may, in fact, endanger human pregnancies.

Inflammation may also explain another set of findings regarding preterm birth involving the omega-3 fatty acid, DHA. In a study of 291 low-income, pregnant women, participants were randomly assigned to receive either DHA-enriched eggs or regular eggs. They were to consume these daily during the last trimester of their pregnancies. This sample was predominantly African American (73%), a group generally at risk for preterm birth. DHA is a long-chain omega-3 fatty acid with anti-inflammatory effects (these effects are described in more detail in a subsequent section). Even when controlling for confounding factors, women who received the DHA-enriched eggs had an average increase in gestation of six days, $\pm$ 2.3 days (Smuts et al., 2003). The DHA-enriched eggs may have increased gestation length by decreasing inflammation. There were no adverse events for mothers or babies, and compliance rates for the intervention were high.

Not every study has found a relationship between depression and low birth weight or prematurity, however. In a large cohort study of 10,967 women, investigators found that women depressed during pregnancy were significantly more likely to have a low birth weight baby (Evan et al., 2007). However, once the investigators controlled for confounding factors, with smoking being the largest, this relationship disappeared. The authors concluded that there was no independent relationship between depression and low birth weight. However, given that depressed women are more likely to smoke and that depression may mediate smoking, the authors' statement about lack of a relationship may be premature.

Another recent study included three groups: depressed pregnant women who were taking antidepressants (N=49); depressed women not on antidepressants (N=22); and healthy controls (N=19; Suri et al., 2007). The authors concluded that depression did not decrease gestational age— antidepressants did. However, depressed women in both the medication and no-medication groups had high levels of stress and depression. So, we may not be able to conclude from these findings that it was the medications, not stress and depression, which increased risk.

Inflammation may also have a role in a common complication of preterm birth: neonatal jaundice. This study compared 32 full-term neonates with neonatal jaundice to 29 term neonates without jaundice (Zanardo et al., 2007). In this study, mothers of infants with jaundice had significantly higher concentrations of IL-1β in their colostrum than mothers of babies without jaundice. The researchers observed similar trends for IL-6, IL-8, IL-10, and TNF-α. These cytokines correlated significantly with each other, but not with serum bilirubin levels. At this point, it's difficult to know what these findings mean. Could mothers' stress and depression increase breastmilk cytokines—

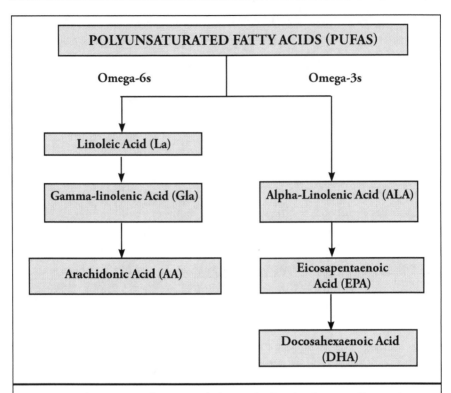

Figure 5: Polyunsaturated Fatty Acids (PUFAs): Omega-6s versus Omega 3s
The essential fatty acids are linoleic acid (omega-6) and α-linolenic acid (omega-3). These are the parent fatty acids. The long-chain omega-3 fatty acids are EPA and DHA, the only omega-3s relevant to depression. The long-chain omega-6 fatty acid is arachidonic acid (Wang *et al.*, 2004).

increasing the risk of jaundice? Could high cytokine levels in colostrum be in response to the neonatal jaundice? Are they unrelated? For now, this remains an intriguing finding, but one future studies should explore in more depth.

In summary, recent studies have implicated inflammation in the etiology of depression. These findings provide a backdrop to understanding non-pharmacologic treatments: omega-3s, bright light therapy, exercise, social support, psychotherapy, and St. John's wort. All are effective, at least in part, because they decrease inflammation. The first modality is omega-3 fatty acids.

OMEGA-3 FATTY ACIDS

What we eat—or don't eat—is likely making us sick. For more than 100 years, an increasing number of people have developed inflammation-related conditions, including heart disease and diabetes. Rates of major depression have followed a similar curve, leading researchers to conclude that these are not independent events (Kiecolt-Glaser *et al.*, 2007). The health impact of Western diets has been observed in a series of epidemiologic studies. The rise in depression and other conditions corresponds to a rather striking change in our diets, specifically regarding our consumption of fats. We now consume more omega-6 fatty acids and fewer omega-3s than we did a century ago. This change has had a major impact on our physical and mental health.

Omega-6s are found in vegetable oils, such as corn and safflower oils, and are a staple of many processed foods. While omega-6s are necessary for good nutrition, they increase inflammation, particularly when we consume too many of them (Kiecolt-Glaser *et al.*, 2007; Parker *et al.*, 2006). In previous centuries, our ratio of omega-6s to omega-3s has been approximately 2 to 3:1. In contrast, the ratio the average North American consumes ranges from 15 to 17:1 (Kiecolt-Glaser *et al.*, 2007).

Omega-3 fatty acids are polyunsaturated fats and are found in plant and marine sources. The parent omega-3 is α-linolenic acid (ALA), and it is found in plants and plant oils, such as walnuts, flax seed, and canola oil. With regard to depression, it is the marine-based, long-chain omega-3 fatty acids that are of interest: eicosapentenoic acid (EPA) and docosahexanoic acid (DHA). A number of recent studies have demonstrated that EPA and DHA are effective for preventing and treating mood disorders. Researchers have documented these effects in population studies, randomized clinical trials, and in prevention studies. These long-chain fatty acids must be consumed as part of our diets because humans cannot convert them from other foods (Parker *et al.*, 2006). Unfortunately, the diets of many living in Western industrialized countries are deficient in both. For example, in a nationally representative U.S. sample, only 25% of the population reported consuming any EPA or DHA in the previous 24 hours (Wang *et al.*, 2004).

EPA and DHA appear to have different functions in maintaining mental health. DHA is found in the non-myelin cell membranes of the central nervous system. High concentrations of DHA are found in the synaptic membranes,

Table 1: Dietary Sources of Polyunsaturated Fatty Acids (PUFAs)			
Omega 6 Fatty Acids	Dietary Sources	Omega 3 Fatty Acids	Dietary Sources
Linoleic Acid (LA) 18:2 n-6	Sunflower, soy, cottonseed, safflower oils	Alpha-Linolenic acid (ALA) 18:3 n-3	Canola, soybean, flaxseed oils, grains, green vegetables, flax seed, walnuts
Gamma-Linolenic Acid (GLA) 18:3 n-6	Evening primrose, borage, black currant oils	Eicosapentaenoic acid (EPA) 20:5 n-3	Fish liver oils, fish eggs
Arachidonic acid (AA) 20:4 n-6	Animal fats, brain, organ meats, egg yolk	Docosahexaenoic Acid (DHA) 22:6 n-3	Human milk, egg yolks, fish liver oils, fish eggs, liver, brain, other organ meats
Source: Wang *et al.*, 2004.			

and it appears to have a critical role in synaptic transmission and membrane fluidity. DHA can also improve depression by stopping depression's inhibition of neurogenesis of the hippocampus. EPA decreases inflammatory eicosanoids, which includes prostaglandins, leukotrienes, and thromboxanes, because it competes with proinflammatory arachidonic acid for the same metabolic pathways. EPA also inhibits production of proinflammatory cytokines (Jensen, 2006; Rees *et al.*, 2005).

The Mental Health Effects of EPA and DHA in Population Studies

Researchers first documented the mental-health effects of EPA/DHA via population studies. Specifically, researchers compared national rates of fish consumption with rates of depression and other affective disorders across different countries (Kiecolt-Glaser *et al.*, 2007; Maes & Smith, 1998). Several recent studies have found that populations who eat more fatty, coldwater fish have higher levels of EPA and DHA and lower rates of affective disorders. Summarizing these studies, Parker and colleagues (2006) noted a surprisingly low incidence of seasonal depression in places where researchers would expect to find it (e.g., Iceland, Finland, Japan). These findings were likely due to the high amounts of fish consumed. Kiecolt-Glaser *et al.* (2007) also noted that depression is 10 times more common in countries where people don't eat fish—or eat a small amount of it.

In a study of 3,204 adults from Finland, researchers assessed depression via the Beck Depression Inventory and frequency of fish consumption via questionnaire (Tanskanen *et al.*, 2001). Using multiple logistic regression, the authors found that depressive symptoms were more likely in participants who ate smaller amounts of fish. Even after controlling for possible confounders— such as smoking, infrequent exercise, and unemployment—the likelihood of being depressed was 31% higher among individuals who did not eat high amounts of seafood.

Noaghiul and Hibbeln (2003) noted that rates of bipolar disorders were lower in countries where people ate a large amount of fish. In their study, they merged mental health data from the 10-nation Cross-National Collaborative Group with national fish consumption data from the World Health Organization. Using logarithmic regression models, they found that greater fish consumption predicted lower rates of bipolar I disorder, bipolar II disorder, and bipolar spectrum disorder. They noted that the strongest findings were for bipolar II disorder, which has prominent depressive symptoms. The authors concluded that while they could not establish a causal relationship, their findings were consistent with deficiencies in omega-3s being related to higher risk for mental disorders.

Fish consumption has a similar effect on postpartum depression. Rees and colleagues (2005) observed that the rates for postpartum depression in North America and Europe are 10 times those in Taiwan, Japan, Hong Kong, and some regions of China. In a large population study with more than 14,000 women from 22 countries, Hibbeln (2002) noted that postpartum depression was up to 50 times more common in countries with low fish consumption. For example, the rate of postpartum depression in Singapore was 0.5%. In South Africa, it was 24.5%. Mothers who ate high amounts of seafood during pregnancy and who had high levels of DHA in their milk postpartum had lower rates of postpartum depression. Rates of postpartum depression were not related to levels of EPA or arachidonic acid (a proinflammatory omega-6).

Omega-3 status has also been related to suicide attempts. In this study, 33 patients who were depressed, but not on medications, were monitored for

19

suicide attempts over a two-year period (Sublette *et al.*, 2006). The researchers assessed plasma polyunsaturated fatty acid levels at the beginning of follow-up. Seven patients attempted suicide, and two fatty acid levels predicted attempts: low DHA and a high ratio of omega-6s to omega-3s. Neither arachidonic acid nor EPA levels predicted suicide attempts.

Not all researchers have found that lower rates of depression correspond to fish consumption, however. In a study of 865 pregnant Japanese women, investigators failed to find lower rates of depression in women who ate more fish (Miyake *et al.*, 2006). Specifically, they found no dose-response effect of fish intake, EPA, DHA, omega-6s, or ratio of omega-6s to omega-3s on postpartum depression. There are some limitations of these findings, however. First, fatty acid levels were not assessed directly, but estimated from a dietary questionnaire administered during pregnancy. Second, the population they assessed has one of the highest fish-consumption rates in the world. It's possible that the researchers encountered a ceiling effect because none of the women were deficient—so it may have been difficult to observe differences between the groups. In addition, depression was assessed anywhere between 2 and 9 months postpartum. That wide range could have influenced the findings, as rates of depression vary by when in the postpartum period they are collected. Having a seven-month assessment period could have obscured their findings.

In summary, eating fish appears to have a beneficial effect on men and women's mental health. Noaghiul and Hibbeln (2003) noted that countries where people ate less than 50 pounds of seafood a year (1 to 1.5 pounds per person per week) had the highest rates of affective disorders. This finding provides some guidance about how much people need to eat to avoid being deficient.

Treatment with EPA and DHA

The effects of EPA/DHA have also been observed using fish-oil supplements. Treatment studies specifically add an active substance to a treatment and assess its results. In the clinical trials of EPA/DHA, researchers gave either a placebo, EPA alone, or EPA/DHA supplements to people with affective disorders (Parker *et al.*, 2006; Peet & Stokes, 2005). Investigators have generally found that EPA is the most effective omega-3 for treating depression. When EPA was added to patients' medications, they were significantly less depressed than those who received medication and a placebo. EPA has also been used as a mono-treatment (Peet & Horrobin, 2002; Peet &

Stokes, 2005).

In a study of 20 patients with major depression, patients were randomized to receive either ethyl-EPA (2 g a day) or a placebo in addition to their regular antidepressant medications (Nemets *et al.*, 2002). By the third week of the study, patients who received EPA were significantly less depressed.

EPA and DHA have also been used as a monotherapy for depression. In a study of 28 children, ages 6 to 12 with major depressive disorder, children who received 400 mg EPA and 200 mg DHA had significantly improved depression compared with children who received a placebo (Nemets *et al.*, 2006). The children were assessed at baseline, and at 2, 4, 8, 12, and 16 weeks. By one month, 7 out of 10 children in the EPA/DHA group had a 50% reduction in their depression. There were no adverse effects noted.

EPA also helped treat the depression in bipolar disorder in a 12-week double-blind trial in London (Frangou *et al.*, 2006). In this study, 75 patients were randomly assigned to one of three conditions for adjunctive therapy: placebo, 1 gram ethyl-EPA, or 2 grams ethyl-EPA. Both EPA groups showed substantial improvement after 12 weeks over the placebo. A dose of 1 gram was as effective as 2 grams, and there was no advantage to 2 grams over 1 gram. Depression was measured by the Hamilton Rating Scale for Depression and the Clinical Global Impression scale. Summarizing their findings, the authors noted that EPA was well-tolerated and safe, that it had an antidepressant effect, and that it may prove more acceptable to patients than pharmacologic interventions.

EPA/DHA have also been helpful with other emotional states. Hallahan and colleagues (2007) tested the efficacy of EPA/DHA supplementation in patients with recurrent self-harm. In this study, 49 patients with repeated acts of self-harm were randomized to receive a placebo or 1.2 grams EPA and 900 mg DHA. After 12 weeks, the patients receiving EPA/DHA had significantly improved depressive symptoms, suicidality, and daily stresses. The authors noted that these were significant markers for suicidality and that supplementation with EPA/DHA had lowered their risk.

These same researchers examined the relationship between EPA/DHA levels and self-harm with another sample (Garland *et al.*, 2007). Their sample included 40 patients who were admitted to the emergency department for self-harm and who met the inclusion criteria (including no current comorbid psychiatric disorder and eating fish no more than once a week). The control group was 27 patients recruited from the medical day ward. Subjects from the control group were also excluded if they ate fish more than once a week. The researchers found that patients with self-harm had significantly lower cholesterol and plasma EPA/DHA levels than healthy controls. In addition, patients with self-harm were higher on all measures of pathology, including depression, impulsivity, and alcohol use. Platelet serotonin levels did not account for these differences.

EPA was also an effective monotherapy in a double-blind, placebo trial for women with borderline personality disorder (Zanarini & Frankenburg, 2003). In this study, 30 women with borderline personality disorder were randomly assigned to receive either 1 gram of EPA or a placebo for eight weeks of treatment (N=20 in EPA group, N=10 in the placebo group). At the end of the study, those receiving EPA were significantly less aggressive and depressed than those in the placebo group.

Not all studies have found that EPA/DHA are effective treatments, however. A recent open-label trial with mothers who had had previous episodes of postpartum depression found that fish oil supplements did not prevent depression from occurring after a subsequent delivery. In this study, women were recruited between 34 to 36 weeks gestation. The women were treated through 12 weeks postpartum, with dosages of 1,730 mg EPA and 1,230 mg DHA. When four of the seven women recruited for the study became depressed, recruitment ceased. The authors hypothesized several possible explanations for their findings, including an inadequate dose of EPA or DHA, administration that was too late in the pregnancy to prevent depression, and the wrong ratio of EPA to DHA. Even with their findings, however, the authors indicated that the results of other studies support continued investigation of EPA and DHA in the treatment of postpartum mood disorders (Marangell *et al.*, 2004).

In summary, an expert panel of the American Psychiatric Association recently concluded that EPA was a promising treatment for mood disorders and that it can used alone or in combination with DHA and/or medications

Table 2: Dosages of EPA/DHA
200-400 mg DHA for prevention of depression
1,000 mg EPA for treatment of depression (with medication and/or DHA)
U.S. Food and Drug Administration GRAS (generally recognized as safe)
Levels: 1500 mg DHA
3000 mg DHA/EPA

(Freeman *et al.*, 2006a). Peet and Stokes' (2005) review found that 1 gram of EPA per day was the effective dose for treatment. Doses higher than 2 grams seemed to have the reverse effect and actually increased depressive symptoms. DHA alone is not an effective treatment for depression (Akabas *et al.*, 2006), but it can be used in addition to EPA. **Table 2** lists current recommended dosages for EPA and DHA.

The Anti-Inflammatory Effects of EPA and DHA

The above-cited studies indicate that EPA and DHA have a role in the prevention and treatment of postpartum depression. The intriguing question is why. It wasn't until recently that researchers confirmed what they suspected: that EPA and DHA are anti-inflammatory (Peet & Stokes, 2005).

In a large population study (N=1,123), high levels of EPA and DHA were related to lower levels of proinflammatory cytokines (IL-1α, IL-1β, IL-6, and TNF-α) and higher levels of anti-inflammatory cytokines, such as IL-10. For people with low levels of EPA and DHA, the opposite was true: they had high levels of proinflammatory cytokines and low levels of anti-inflammatory cytokines (Ferrucci *et al.*, 2006). This study had several advantages over previous research. The sample in this study was representative of the population—not a specific subgroup. The fatty acids were directly measured in the plasma rather than estimated from patient dietary reports. It was the first study that specifically examined the relationship between fatty acids and cytokines.

Inflammatory eicosanoids are also higher in depressed patients than their non-depressed counterparts (Parker *et al.*, 2006). Eicosanoids are derived from high levels of arachidonic acid—an omega-6. Arachidonic acid and EPA compete for enzymes responsible for eicosanoid formation. Higher levels of EPA inhibit both the production of eicosanoids and the proinflammatory cytokines IL-1β, IL-6, IFN-γ, and TNF-α—the very ones implicated in depression (Jensen, 2006; Parker *et al.*, 2006; Peet & Stokes, 2005).

Kiecolt-Glaser and colleagues (2007) noted that inflammation levels are lower in patients with either high levels of omega-3s or a lower ratio of omega-6s to omega-3s. In their study of older adults, depression and a high ratio of omega-6s to omega-3s dramatically increased levels of proinflammatory cytokines (IL-6 & TNF-s). A high ratio of omega-6s to omega-3s indicates an omega-3 deficiency. Patients who were both depressed and had low levels of omega-3s had the highest levels of proinflammatory cytokines. The authors noted that a diet that is low in EPA/DHA increases the risk of both depression and other diseases related to chronic inflammation.

One study, however, found that neither EPA nor DHA had an impact on proinflammatory cytokines (Kew et al., 2004). In this study, 42 healthy adults were randomly assigned to receive EPA (4.7 g), DHA (4.9 g), or a placebo. Supplementation with EPA or DHA significantly altered the fatty acid composition of the plasma phospholipids and neutrophil lipids. Neither altered the production of TNF-α, IL-10, IL-6, or IL-1β. The authors noted that their findings contradicted earlier findings with smaller dosages. A study by these same investigators, with a sample of 150 healthy men and women, found that EPA/DHA (1.7 g) or ALA (9.5 g) did not alter immune function. The immune parameters they examined included proinflammatory cytokines and the percentage of monocytes engaged in phagocytosis. They noted that supplementation with EPA and DHA did not have a harmful effect on immunologic function and concluded that recommended guidelines could be increased without any harmful effects on the immune system (Kew et al., 2003).

What these conflicting findings might reveal is that smaller dosages are more effective in treating mood disorders than large doses. Indeed, as described above, a review of EPA as a treatment for depression revealed that dosages larger than 2 grams were related to higher levels of depression (Peet & Stokes, 2005). Kew and colleagues' (2003; 2004) findings are consistent with that. This could also mean that supplementation does not harmfully alter immune parameters, but may indeed modulate immune function, so that it is functioning well, but not excessively.

EPA/DHA and the Stress Response

Researchers have examined another aspect of EPA/DHA that is relevant to our discussion of postpartum depression: the impact of EPA and DHA on stress. More specifically, do EPA and DHA have an adaptogenic role in stress by regulating and attenuating the stress response? Several studies have suggested that they may indeed. When college students had a high ratio of omega-6s to omega-3s, they had more inflammation when exposed to a lab-induced stressor. In contrast, students with higher levels of EPA/DHA had a lower inflammatory response to stress (Maes et al., 2000).

Similarly, Kiecolt-Glaser and colleagues (2007) noted that previous stress and depression appear to "prime" the inflammatory response, and that subsequent stressors led to substantial increases in inflammation. What's more concerning is that chronic stress impacts both acute and chronic production of proinflammatory cytokines. The good news is that EPA/DHA supplementation seemed to halt that process and its maladaptive impact on mood. In their study of 43 older adults, they noted that "even modest supplementation with n-3 PUFAs (omega-3 polyunsaturated fatty acids) reduces plasma norepinephrine, an important link to the stress response" (p. 221).

Another study in Japan had similar findings while investigating the impact of EPA/DHA supplementation on 21 young adults (Hamazaki *et al.*, 2005). In a double-blind trial, participants took either a placebo or 762 mg of EPA/DHA for two months. The researchers noted that EPA concentrations increased in the red blood cell membranes in the supplemented group. The EPA/DHA group also had significantly decreased levels of plasma norepinephrine.

Some parallel work has been done with regard to Type 2 diabetes. In a review, Delarue and colleagues (2004) found that in healthy patients, fish oil reduced insulin resistance and plasma triglycerides and increased resilience to stress by decreasing the activity of the sympathetic nervous system. Fish oil did not reduce insulin resistance in patients with diabetes, but did lower triglycerides. The authors concluded that fish oil showed promise in the prevention of insulin resistance and related health problems.

Not all researchers have found that EPA/DHA attenuate stress beyond the placebo effect, however. In a study of high-stress individuals, researchers randomized participants into one of three groups: no treatment, placebo, or fish oil (Bradbury *et al.*, 2005). The placebo group received 6 grams per day of olive oil. The treatment group received 6 grams of tuna oil, which contained 1.5 grams DHA and 360 mg EPA. Compared to the no-treatment group, perceived stress dropped significantly for the EPA/DHA group. There was, however, no significant difference between the placebo and treatment groups. Although the researchers concluded that their findings support the protective or adaptogenic role for omega-3s in stress, their findings may not support this conclusion, given the large placebo effect and the lack of significant differences between it and findings for the treatment group. One possible limitation in this study was that the investigators used a relatively small dosage of EPA. EPA is likely the fatty acid that lowers stress because it lowers levels of proinflammatory cytokines, prostaglandins, and eicosanoids.

DHA in the Perinatal Period

As described earlier, in Western cultures, pregnant women's diets are often deficient in both EPA and DHA. Writing about mothers in Australia, Rees and colleagues (2005) noted that Australian mothers consume about 15 mg a day. In contrast, Japanese, Koreans, and Norwegians consume about 1,000 mg a day. During the last trimester of pregnancy, babies accumulate an average of 67 mg a day of DHA, so many Australian mothers fall short of what they need. This is true in other Western cultures as well. Because babies need DHA for brain and vision development, women's bodies will preferentially divert it to the baby, and the baby will take the DHA it needs from maternal stores. With each subsequent pregnancy, mothers are further depleted (Freeman et al., 2006b), and mothers' deficiency increases their risk for depression. In the Adelaide Mothers' and Babies' Iron Trial, a 1% increase in plasma DHA was related to a 59% decrease in depressive symptoms postpartum (Rees et al., 2005).

As noted earlier, Hibbeln's (2002) population study found that mothers who had eaten high amounts of seafood during pregnancy and who had high levels of DHA in their milk postpartum had lower levels of postpartum depression. He did not find the same preventative effect for EPA.

DHA may have another effect that could help prevent depression postpartum. In a study of infant sleep, mothers with high levels of DHA during pregnancy had babies who exhibited more mature sleep patterns in the first few days of life. With a sample of 17 neonates, the investigators examined the ratio of quiet to active sleep using a monitor placed beneath the crib mattress. A higher percentage of quiet sleep is characteristic of older babies and an indicator of more mature sleep. Babies whose mothers had high levels of DHA during pregnancy exhibited more mature sleep patterns as neonates. The investigators concluded that babies of high-DHA mothers had more mature central nervous systems than babies of mothers who were low in DHA. Although a small sample, the findings are intriguing. Babies with more mature sleep patterns allow their mothers to get more uninterrupted sleep—and this could have an indirect effect on maternal mental health (Cheruku et al., 2002).

Not every study has found that DHA prevents depression. One-hundred thirty-eight mothers were randomly assigned to receive 200 mg DHA or a placebo for the first four months postpartum (Llorente *et al.*, 2003). The outcome variables studied were plasma phospholipid DHA content, self-reported and syndromal depression, and maternal information processing. Blood was drawn at 37 to 38 weeks gestation and at four months postpartum. Depression was measured by Beck Depression Inventory at baseline, three weeks, and two and four months postpartum. They found that while phospholipid DHA was 50% higher in the supplemented group at four months, DHA did not prevent depression. They found no adverse effects of DHA supplementation for either mother or baby.

The current recommended minimum intake of DHA is 200 to 400 mg a day. This may prove to be a fairly conservative amount—especially given that most women in Western cultures are deficient (see **Table 2**). But for now, this is the consensus recommended amount (Jensen, 2006).

Possible Teratogenicity During Pregnancy and Lactation

One concern about any type of supplementation is whether it's safe for pregnant and breastfeeding women. Most recent studies of either pregnant or breastfeeding women have noted no teratogenic effects with a wide range of dosages (Marangell *et al.*, 2004; Shoji *et al.*, 2006; Smuts *et al.*, 2003). A few studies have found some mild negative effects with very high dosages. These findings are summarized below.

Studies During Pregnancy

Most studies of pregnant women and EPA/DHA are population studies examining fish or fish-oil consumption. One study sampled 182 women from the Faroe Islands: a community between Shetland and Iceland (Grandjean *et al.*, 2001). The average fish consumption in this sample was 72 grams of fish, 12 grams of whale muscle, and 7 grams of blubber a day. The researchers found that DHA was the best predictor of gestational length, with a 1% increase in relative concentration related to a 1.5 day increase in gestation. However, an increase of 1% in relative EPA concentration was related to a 246 gram decrease in birthweight. This effect was independent of the effects of environmental contaminants. It should be noted that this was a very large dose.

Another study of 488 women in Iceland found that the odds ratio for developing hypertension in pregnancy was 4.7 for women taking cod liver oil (Olafsdottir *et al.*, 2006). There are some methodologic issues to consider with this sample, however, as we interpret the findings. First, cod liver oil contains not only EPA and DHA, but three fat-soluble vitamins (A, D, and E) that can be toxic in large doses. Levels of these vitamins could influence their findings. For example, the researchers noted that a higher intake of Vitamin D increased the likelihood of hypertensive disorders in pregnancy. Second, consumption of cod liver oil was estimated from questionnaire data—not directly measured in participant serum. Third, when data were divided into centiles, the authors noted a u-shaped curve, with the odds ratios of hypertension being the lowest for those with a modest supplementation of EPA/DHA, similar to findings of other studies. Their findings suggest that modest amounts of EPA/DHA (0.1 to 0.9 g) appear safe with no increased risk to the mother or baby, but higher amounts could be a problem.

A large, European multi-site study examined the prophylactic and therapeutic role of fish oil in women who had experienced preterm delivery (N=232), intrauterine growth retardation (IUGR; N=280), or pregnancy induced hypertension (N=386) during a previous pregnancy (Olsen *et al.*, 2000). Women were randomized to receive 2.7 grams fish oil (1.3 g EPA, .9 g DHA), 6.1 grams fish oil (2.9 g EPA, 2.1 g DHA), or an olive-oil placebo. For women in both fish-oil groups, recurrence risk for preterm labor dropped from 33% to 21%, but birth weight also dropped in the fish-oil groups. Fish oil had no impact on IUGR or pregnancy-induced hypertension. Seven of the women receiving fish oil and three who received olive oil had infants with intracranial hemorrhage. The authors noted that this number was consistent with a chance finding. Nevertheless, they recommended monitoring women taking fish oil at the end of pregnancy. Note that these were high dosages in both conditions, perhaps a lower dose is advisable. There was no difference between the fish-oil and olive-oil groups for other neonatal complications.

A randomized trial of 341 women compared cod liver oil supplementation (803 mg EPA, 1,183 mg DHA) to corn oil from 18 weeks gestation to three months postpartum (Hellend *et al.*, 2003). All the babies in this study breastfed for at least three months. There were no teratogenic effects noted. At four years of age, children whose mothers had taken cod liver oil during pregnancy and lactation had a higher Mental Processing Composite score. This score correlated with head circumference at birth, but not birth weight or gestational age. Only pregnancy intake of DHA was significantly related to mental abilities at age four.

Another study examined the effect of supplementation of 150 mg EPA and 500 mg DHA from 20 weeks gestation to delivery (Shoji *et al.*, 2006). There were 46 pregnant women in the study. The researchers were testing whether DHA enhanced oxidative stress because of the increased likelihood of lipid peroxidation. Women were assessed at 20 and 30 weeks gestation and at delivery. The researchers found no adverse effects and concluded that 500 mg of DHA and 150 mg EPA did not enhance lipid peroxidation or oxidative DNA damage.

A clinical trial (Malcolm *et al.*, 2003) randomly assigned 100 mothers to either fish oil (200 mg DHA) or a placebo from 15 weeks gestation to delivery. Fatty acids were measured in plasma and red blood cells at 15, 28, and 40 weeks, and in umbilical cord blood. Infant visual evoked potentials were measured at birth and at 50 and 66 weeks. Interestingly, there was no impact of maternal supplementation on level of DHA in umbilical cord blood or visual evoked potentials. However, infant DHA status (regardless of group) did make a difference. High-DHA infants showed increased maturation of the central visual pathways. The authors noted that their findings suggested that infants accrue sufficient amounts, in spite of and/or at the expense of their mothers to meet the needs of their developing neural and visual systems. They noted no teratogenic effects of supplementation.

Impact on Breastfeeding

EPA/DHA also appear to have no negative impact on breastfeeding babies, even at relatively high dosages. Freeman and colleagues (2006b) conducted a small, randomized trial using three different dosages of EPA/DHA with 16 mothers with postpartum major depression (300 mg EPA/200 mg DHA; 840 mg EPA/560 mg DHA; or 1,680 mg EPA; 1,120 mg DHA). They noted that depression significantly decreased in all three groups. The study was limited by a small sample and no control group (therefore, not ruling out a placebo effect). There were no negative effects noted for mother or baby.

Hawkes and colleagues (2002) conducted a double-blind trial with women who were three days postpartum. Women received either a placebo, 700 mg EPA/300 mg DHA, or 140 mg EPA/600 mg DHA for twelve weeks. Supplementation with EPA/DHA did not alter cytokine levels in breastmilk. There was no change in mean rank concentrations of IL-6 or TNF-α in the aqueous phase of the milk, nor were there any correlations between the milk DHA, EPA, or cytokine concentration. The authors concluded that these levels of supplementation did not cause perturbations in cytokine concentrations and were thus safe for breastfeeding women, without harm to the baby.

At very high dosages of EPA/DHA supplementation, researchers have had concerns about possible changes in breastmilk fatty acid composition. In one study where 83 mothers were supplemented from 20 weeks gestation to delivery, there were significant changes in fatty acid composition of breastmilk. But these changes may, indeed, prove beneficial—not harmful. Fish oil supplementation significantly increased EPA and DHA concentrations in breastmilk (Dunstan *et al.*, 2004a), and in the erythrocytes of mothers and babies in the fish-oil group (Dunstan *et al.*, 2004b). There were no differences between the treatment and control groups in three immune parameters in breastmilk: IL-6, IL-10, and IL-13. But, higher levels of EPA/DHA were related to increased levels of two other immune parameters: IgA and sCD14. The researchers identified these higher levels as potentially protective. The dosage used in this study was very high (2.2 g DHA, 1.5 g EPA): 11 times the recommended minimum of DHA. Even with this large dose, EPA/DHA might help promote beneficial probiotic Lactobacilli, which can help protect against the development of allergic disease.

Dunstan and colleagues did express some concerns about what the alterations in fatty acid composition might mean. One concern they raised is that EPA lowers arachidonic acid levels, and they indicated that we needed more information before making dietary recommendations (Dunstan *et al.*, 2004b). Even with these cautions in place, however, it should be noted again that the levels of supplementation they used in their study were much higher than recommended. Even at this high dosage, the cautions they raised were hypothetical, rather than observed effects.

Sources of EPA and DHA

Fish is the most common dietary source of EPA and DHA. Unfortunately, pregnant or breastfeeding women often need to limit the amount of fish they eat because of contaminants in seafood. Fortunately, there are alternative sources of EPA and DHA that are tested for contaminants and are contaminant free. Fish oil is one important source. The U.S. Pharmacopeia is an independent, not-for-profit organization that tests and verifies brands of supplements—including fish oil. Companies can submit to voluntary testing to be USP verified. The USP rigorously tests for contaminants and lists specific brand names that they verify on their Web site (www.USP.org). Other sources of DHA include prenatal vitamins and fortified foods. Some of these sources of DHA are vegetarian and kosher. Be sure to read labels of fortified foods carefully, however. Some advertise "omega-3s" and contain flax, not EPA/DHA. These products are not harmful, but they won't help with depression. There is currently no vegetarian source of EPA; fish or fish oil are the only sources. **Table 3** lists sources of EPA/DHA that are safe for pregnant and breastfeeding women.

Table 3: Sources of Contaminant-Free EPA/DHA*
Pharmaceutical-Grade Fish Oil (EPA & DHA)
Carlson Labs (www.CarlsonLabs.com)
Vital Nutrients (www.VitalNutrients.net)
Brands of Over-the-Counter Fish-Oil Supplements verified by the U.S. Pharmacopeia (www.usp.org)
Berkley & Jensen, Equaline, Kirkland Signature, Nature Made, NutriPlus
Vegetarian DHA Supplements
Nature's Way DHA (www.NaturesWay.com)
O-mega-Zen-3 (www.Nutru.com)
Prenatal Supplements with DHA
OptiNate (First Horizons Pharmaceutical)
Citracal Prenatal + DHA (Mission Pharmacal)
DHA-Fortified Foods
DHA-fortified eggs (Gold Circle Farms)
Oh Mama! Nutrition bar for pregnant and breastfeeding women
Odwalla Soymilk
Silk Soymilk with DHA (small amount)
Bellybar Nutrition Bar (Nutrabella)Breyer's Yogurt with DHA
* The author has no financial relationship to any of these companies.

What About Flax Seed?

For people who do not want to take fish oil, many have turned to flax seed as an alternative. The principal omega-3 in flaxseed is alpha-linolenic acid (ALA). As described earlier, ALA is an essential fatty acid and is the parent omega-3 fatty acid. Although our body can convert ALA to EPA and DHA, it does so inefficiently (see Figure 1); only 10% to 15% of ALA is converted to EPA and DHA (Parker *et al.*, 2006). Supplementation with ALA does not increase EPA and DHA levels and has no impact on depression (Bratman & Girman, 2003; Caughey *et al.* 1996; Kew *et al.*, 2003). Flax seed does, however, have cardiovascular benefits and is not harmful. It simply does not prevent or treat depression.

Remaining Questions

Although there is a large amount of evidence that supports use of EPA/ DHA, Parker and colleagues (2006) noted that a number of questions remain. First, does supplementation with omega-3s, particularly EPA, have the greatest potential if used by itself or as an augmentative therapy to antidepressants? What constitutes the optimum amount, and more importantly, what constitutes a deficiency? What ratio of DHA to EPA is optimal? And what is the optimal ratio of omega-6s to omega-3s? A related question is whether the ratio is important, or whether this question becomes moot once the deficiency of omega-3 is addressed? Finally, how long must women be supplemented before their deficiency is corrected? Unfortunately, we do not have answers to these questions yet. But data suggests that the ratio of omega-6s to omega-3s is likely less important once the deficiency in omega-3s is addressed. And, at least we have a starting place for recommending how much women should take of both DHA and EPA.

Summary

Increasing evidence suggests that DHA can help prevent depression in new mothers and that EPA is a useful treatment—alone or in combination with medications and/or DHA. EPA and DHA also appear to be helpful in the treatment of other affective disorders, including bipolar disorder, borderline personality, and suicide risk. A review in the British Journal of Psychiatry summarized these findings as follows:

> There is good evidence that psychiatric illness is associated with the depletion of EFAs [essential fatty acids] and, crucially, that supplementation can result in clinical amelioration....The clinical trial data may herald a simple, safe and effective adjunct to our standard

treatments (Hallahan & Garland, 2005, p. 276).

EPA and DHA are one promising intervention for mothers, and risk for either pregnant or breastfeeding women appear only at dosages well above the recommended amounts. The next modality—bright light therapy—has similar benefits with few apparent negative side effects.

BRIGHT LIGHT THERAPY

Some people in northern latitudes dread the change of seasons. Shorter, darker days mean fatigue, oversleeping, eating too many carbohydrates, and having a general sense of malaise: a pattern known as seasonal affective disorder (SAD; Sullivan & Paynes, 2007). In the Northern Hemisphere, seasonal affective disorder is depression that occurs during late fall and winter months, as darkness occurs earlier in the day. Symptoms include depression, lethargy, difficulty waking, impaired concentration, lack of interest in social activities, and craving carbohydrates, which often leads to winter weight gain (NAMI, 2007).

In a study of 93 Midwestern undergraduates, seasonal affective disorder was much more prevalent than major depression, 28% versus 9% for SAD and major depression, respectively (Sullivan & Payne, 2007). The gender differences in this study were also striking: 42% of women and 11% of men had seasonal affective disorder. Depending on where you live, the results from this study suggest that seasonal depression may be even more likely than major depression in many parts of the world. Fortunately, safe treatments for pregnant and breastfeeding women are available.

For more than 20 years, clinicians have used bright light therapy to successfully treat seasonal affective disorder. Light therapy is another non-pharmacologic treatment that can provide relief within days (NAMI, 2007). Researchers have recently discovered that light therapy is also helpful for other affective disorders, including non-seasonal depression, antenatal and postpartum depression, bipolar disorder, some eating disorders, and certain sleep disorders (Oren et al., 2002; Terman & Terman, 2005). An expert panel for the American Psychiatric Association concluded that bright light therapy was an effective treatment for both seasonal and non-seasonal depression, "with effect sizes equivalent to those in most antidepressant pharmacotherapy trials" (Golden et al., 2005, p. 656). The effect sizes ranged from 0.84 for reduction of symptoms, 0.73 for use of dawn simulation in seasonal affective disorder, and 0.53 for treatment of non-seasonal depression.

Light Therapy in Seasonal Depression

In a recent clinical trial, patients were randomized to receive either light therapy at 10,000 lux for 30 minutes a day and a placebo medication or 100 lux (placebo light) with 20 mg fluoxetine (Lam *et al.*, 2006). A total of 96 patients with seasonal major depression participated for eight weeks. The researchers found that light therapy was as effective as fluoxetine in relieving symptoms: the clinical response rate was 67% for both groups. By one week, patients in the light-therapy group had a greater response to treatment, but this difference disappeared at subsequent assessment points. There were more side effects with fluoxetine, but both treatments were generally well-tolerated, with no overall difference in adverse effects. The researchers conducted a separate analysis for the most severely depressed patients. They found that fluoxetine and bright light were both effective for severe depression, but there was no significant differences between the groups - bright light and medications were equally effective.

To date, only a few studies have included pregnant and postpartum women. Their findings have been mixed in terms of effectiveness. For example, bright light was helpful in two case studies of new mothers who suddenly became depressed after the birth of their babies (Corral *et al.*, 2000). These mothers refused antidepressants, but agreed to a trial of bright light therapy. Both of these women responded to bright light therapy and had significantly lower rates of depressive symptoms after treatment.

In a recent study of 15 women with postpartum depression, 10 were assigned to receive light at 10,000 lux for six weeks and five were assigned to dim red light (600 lux). After six weeks, both groups improved, and there was no significant difference between the groups (Corral *et al.*, 2007). Another study, an open-label trial with 16 pregnant women with major depression, found that there was a 49% improvement in depressive symptoms after three weeks of treatment with bright light (10,000 lux). Based on their results, the authors recommended a randomized trial to further test the efficacy of this intervention with pregnant women (Oren *et al.*, 2002).

Light Intensity, Duration, and Timing of Light Exposure

Light intensity also appears to influence treatment effectiveness. Researchers have investigated a wide range of intensities—and several appear effective. Light is measured in units of lumen and lux. Lumen refers to how bright the light is. Lux refers to lumen over a certain area. Even with the same lumen, light spread over a wider area would have lower lux. By way of comparison, 400 lux is the approximate amount of light in a brightly lit office, while 32,000 lux is the brightness of sunlight on an average day. With regard to bright light therapy, lights with intensities of 10,000 lux appear most effective. At this level of intensity, 30 to 40 minutes of exposure is sufficient. Two studies with light exposures of 30 to 40 minutes at 10,000 lux achieved a 75% remission rate in depression. It took two hours to achieve similar remission rates at 2,500 lux. And in some cases, even with longer exposure, lower-intensity lights were not as effective (Terman & Terman, 2005). Another problem with longer exposure times is that patients are less likely to comply. This may be particularly true for mothers of young children who probably won't find it practical to sit in front of a light box for two or three hours.

Another study used a Litebook LED (1,350 lux) for 30 minutes and found that the amount of light significantly lowered depression scores compared to a placebo light (Desan et al., 2007). This was a small trial with 26 participants (23 completed the study). Patients were assessed after one, two, three, and fours weeks of treatment. By four weeks, 57% of patients in the LED condition were in remission compared to 11% of patients in the control condition. The authors speculated that this lower intensity light worked because it was in the 450-480 nm range and that melatonin rhythms were best shifted by those wavelengths. Because of this concentration in short wavelengths, even lower intensity light might prove as effective as brighter light boxes, while using smaller, more convenient devices.

Timing

Timing of light exposure also makes a difference. Morning exposure to bright light is generally more successful than light exposure later in the day. In their review, Terman and Terman (2005) cited one analysis of 332 patients across 25 different studies that compared administration of light in the morning, mid-day, and evening. They noted remission rates after one week of treatment, with significantly higher rates in the morning (53%), compared with mid-day (32%) and evening (38%) exposures. According to their analysis, morning light should be administered 8.5 hours after a patient's melatonin onset. Melatonin onset can be difficult—or impractical—to assess directly. However, the Center for Environmental Therapeutics (www.cet.org) has a free online questionnaire to help patients estimate this and calculate individual treatment time.

One exception to the use of morning light is in patients with bipolar disorder. Morning light exposure can increase the risk of a manic episode. This problem can be addressed by timing light exposure to later in the day and having them continue on their medications during light treatment (NAMI, 2007; Terman & Terman, 2005).

Dawn Simulation

Because of the effectiveness of morning light exposure, a variant to standard light therapy has recently been added to the repertoire of possible treatments: dawn simulation. As the name implies, dawn simulation refers to a light that comes on before a patient is awake and gradually increases in intensity over a period of 15 to 90 minutes (the length can be tailored to individual preference). The advantage to this treatment is that it does not require sitting in front of a light box for an extended time, making it a more practical alternative for new mothers or mothers of young children. Although a relatively new technique, it is showing promise as a treatment for seasonal depression (Golden *et al.*, 2005). Some newer lighting devices are both light boxes and dawn simulators.

Dawn simulation specifically addresses the early dawn interval when melatonin levels wane and core body temperature rises. It is during this time when circadian rhythms are most susceptible to light-elicited phase advances. According to this theory, depression is more likely to be triggered when it is still dark outdoors in the early dawn interval. To test this theory, Terman and Terman (2006) randomly assigned 99 adults with seasonal major depression to one of five treatment conditions. These included dawn simulation, dawn light pulse, post-awakening bright light therapy (30 minutes at 10,000 lux), negative air ionization at high flow rate, and ionization at low flow rate. After three weeks of treatment, bright light therapy (57%) and dawn simulation (50%) had the greatest improvement in symptoms. They concluded that bright light therapy still appeared to be the most effective. However, if there are problems with non-compliance or non-response, dawn simulation or dawn pulse were viable alternatives. Recommendations on intensity, timing, and duration of bright light are summarized in **Table 4**.

Table 4: Intensity, Duration and Timing of Bright Light Therapy
• Bright light has been found to be as effective as antidepressants in alleviating seasonal depression.
• 10,000 lux for 30 to 40 minutes is the most commonly used intensity. But lower intensities have also been effective.
• Morning light exposure is more effective than light exposure later in the day.
• Dawn simulation is an alternative to standard light therapy that may prove more practical for mothers of infants or young children.

Why Light is Effective

Researchers have proposed a number of possible mechanisms for why bright light alleviates depression. Most explanations have to do with modifying the internal circadian clock. Exposure to light in dark winter months appears to reset the internal clock.

Our circadian rhythms, or daily patterns of sleep and arousal, are regulated by the pineal gland, which secretes melatonin. The suprachiasmatic nucleus of the hypothalamus regulates synthesis of melatonin (Erman, 2007). The pineal gland responds to light via light receptors in the retina. The superiority of morning-light exposure is likely due to the diurnal variations in retinal photoreceptor sensitivity, with greater sensitivity to morning light. Indeed, exposure to evening light can lead to insomnia and hyperactivation in some people (NAMI, 2007; Terman & Terman, 2005).

Preliminary evidence indicates that there is an inflammatory component to seasonal depression as well. Lam and colleagues (2004) hypothesized that during winter, proinflammatory cytokines increase for patients with seasonal depression. In a study of 15 patients and a matched group of normal controls, those with seasonal affective disorder had significantly higher levels of IL-6. After two weeks of bright light therapy, symptoms improved, and 64% of them had at least a 50% reduction in depressive symptoms. However, light therapy did not alter immune parameters after two weeks. The authors concluded that seasonal depression involves activation of the immune-inflammatory system, which is not immediately altered by light therapy (Leu *et al.*, 2001).

Safety Issues

Because light boxes can be relatively expensive (about $100 U.S.) and appear to be simple, patients often consider assembling a unit themselves. Just because they can, doesn't mean they should. Clinicians generally recommend that patients don't use homemade devices for several reasons having to do with color temperature, another characteristic of light that influences both effectiveness and safety. Color temperature is a characteristic of visible light. The unit of color temperature is kelvin, the spectrum of which ranges from red to violet. The red spectrum is 1800 kelvin and the end of the violet spectrum is 16,000 kelvin. Typical warm daylight ranges from 5000 to 6500 kelvin. In contrast, an incandescent bulb is 2,800 kelvin, which is considerably lower kelvin than daylight.

With color temperature in mind, let's consider the safety of homemade devices. First, it is difficult for consumers to find lights that are of sufficient brightness (lux) to generate a therapeutic effect (despite advertising to the contrary). Second, some patients have experienced excessive irradiation and corneal or eyelid burns with homemade devices. Finally, homemade devices often use incandescent lights. Some of these have been marketed for bright light therapy, but are not recommended because approximately 90% of light output from incandescent bulbs is on the infrared end of the spectrum. Infrared exposure at high intensity can cause damage to the lens, cornea, and retina (Terman & Terman, 2005).

Light boxes with high levels of exposure to UV can also cause eye damage, and there is some controversy about the safety and efficacy of lights that are solely on the blue end of the spectrum. The National Alliance on Mental Illness recommends lights that are encased in a box with a diffusing lens that filters out UV radiation, with a color temperature between 3000 and 6500 degrees Kelvin (NAMI, 2007). These do not harm patients' eyes. "Full spectrum" bulbs are not necessarily an advantage and are often expensive. Patients wanting to try light therapy should use a lighting apparatus from a reputable dealer (see **Table 5** for a listing of possible sources). Since price may be an issue, many hospitals and some manufacturers have loaner programs that allow patients to try the lighting device in their homes before buying them.

Table 5: Resources on Light Therapy
Rosenthal, N.E. (2006). *Winter blues: Everything you need to know to beat seasonal affective disorder, Revised Ed.* New York: Guilford. This book is the "bible" of self-help guides on SAD, written by the physician who first documented the phenomenon. **Center for Environmental Therapeutics** (www.cet.org) CET has a free, online questionnaire to help patients estimate melatonin onset and time their light treatment. **Sources for Light Boxes** The Sunbox Company www.sunbox.com TrueSun.com www.truesun.com

Summary

Bright light therapy is a generally safe, well-tolerated treatment option for seasonal depression. It may relieve non-seasonal depression as well. Bright light therapy is also breastfeeding friendly and can be used during pregnancy. Although therapeutic light boxes can be costly at first, a single purchase will last for years. For patients who dread winter, this investment is often well worth the cost.

EXERCISE

Exercise is another effective treatment for depression in general and postpartum depression in particular (Daley *et al.*, 2007). Traditionally, exercise has been recommended for people with mild-to-moderate depression. But as two clinical trials have found, exercise can also alleviate major depression as effectively as medications. Exercise can also be safely combined with other modalities.

Exercise for Depressed People

Several recent studies have demonstrated that exercise improves mood. Many of these studies are of older adults, who are sometimes at higher risk for depression. Medications can be difficult to manage for this population, as they are frequently taking more than one, so exercise is a good alternative.

In a large population study from Finland (N=3,403), exercise lowered depression and helped with feelings of anger, distrust, and stress. Two to three times a week was enough to achieve this mood-altering effect (Hassmen *et al.*, 2000). Men and women who exercised perceived their health and fitness as better than non-exercisers. Exercise also increased participants' social connections with others.

In a sample of 32 older adults (ages 60 to 84 years), subjects were randomized to one of two conditions: 10 weeks of supervised weight-lifting exercise followed by 10 weeks of unsupervised exercise or attending lectures for 10 weeks (Singh *et al.*, 2001). The patients all had major or minor depression, and the researchers did not contact any study participant until the end of the research period at 26 months. As predicted, the exercise group was significantly less depressed at 20 weeks and at follow-up at 26 months than the non-exercisers. Moreover, at the 26-month follow-up, 33% of the exercisers were still regularly weight lifting versus 0% of the controls.

In a similar study, older adults were randomly assigned to either exercise classes or health education for 10 weeks (Mather *et al.*, 2002). All participants were depressed and on medications, but medications were not adequately controlling their depression. At the end of treatment, 55% of the exercise group was less depressed versus 33% of the education group.

Most of the participants in the previously cited studies had mild-to-moderate depression. But Babyak *et al.'s* (2000) study demonstrated that exercise can be helpful for major depression as well. In this clinical trial, depressed older adults were randomly assigned to one of three groups: exercise alone, sertraline alone, or a combination of exercise and sertraline. After four months, all the patients improved, and there were no differences between the groups. People in the exercise-only group did as well as people in the two medication groups. In addition, people in the exercise-only group were significantly less likely to relapse. Six months after completion of treatment, 28% of the exercise-only group became depressed again versus 51% of the medications-only and medications-exercise groups. The authors concluded that exercise is an effective intervention, even in patients with major depression. Moreover, exercise helps prevent relapse.

This same group of researchers recently replicated their findings (Blumenthal *et al.*, 2007). In the more recent study, 202 adults with major depression were randomized to one of four conditions: sertraline, exercise at home, supervised exercise, or a placebo control. After four months of treatment, 41% of the patients were in remission and no longer met the criteria for major depression. Efficacy rates by treatment were as follows: supervised exercise=45%, home-based exercise=40%, medication=47%, and placebo=31%. The exercise condition was 45 minutes of walking on a treadmill at 70% to 85% maximum heart rate capacity, three times a week for 16 weeks. The home-exercise group received the same instructions, but was not supervised and had minimal contact with the research staff. The authors concluded that the efficacy of exercise was comparable to medications. The supervised program was especially effective, but the home program was also comparable to medications. And all treatments were more effective than the placebo.

The mood-altering effects of exercise appear fairly quickly. In a study of 26 women, Lane and colleagues (2002) measured anger, confusion, depression, fatigue, tension, and vigor before and after two exercise sessions. The women's moods significantly improved after each exercise session. Depressed mood was especially sensitive to exercise and decreased significantly after each session.

Exercise and Inflammation

Exercise works as a treatment for several reasons. It decreases stress and improves self-efficacy, a person's sense of competence and ability to make positive changes in their lives (McAuley et al., 2000). It also influences levels of proinflammatory cytokines as the studies below illustrate. Initially, exercise acts as an acute physical stressor and raises IL-6 and TNF-α. An initial burst of these cytokines does not appear to be harmful. Indeed, and as Goebels and colleagues (2000) point out, in a normally functioning system, high levels of cytokines trigger the body's anti-inflammatory mechanisms to keep inflammation in check.

Over a longer period of time, however, especially in people with chronically elevated proinflammatory cytokines, exercise lowers inflammation. Older adults, for example, are one group with higher levels of proinflammatory cytokines since levels naturally increase as we age. Indeed, researchers hypothesize that this age-related rise in inflammation creates vulnerability to diseases such as heart disease, cancer, and Alzheimer's (Kiecolt-Glaser et al., 2007). Because of this increased vulnerability of older adults, they are frequently the population of choice for studies on exercise, depression, and inflammation. The results of these studies are helpful in understanding the mechanism for exercise's impact on depression.

A study of adults, ages 60 to 90, tested the effect of physical activity on perceived stress, mood, and quality of life. The researchers also assessed serum IL-6 and cortisol. The patients (N=10) assigned to the exercise group were instructed to walk for 30 minutes at a rate that would elevate their heart rate to 60% of its maximal capacity, five times a week for the 10-week study. The control group was 10 older adults who were not engaging in physical activity. After the 10-week exercise intervention, the subjects had significantly lower stress on the Perceived Stress Scale and improved mood and quality of life on the SF-36 Health Questionnaire. They reported better physical functioning, more vitality, better mental health, and less bodily pain. They also had a significant decrease in serum IL-6 (Starkweather, 2007). This effect was independent of an association between psychological variables and IL-6. In others words, depression did not mediate these findings.

Another study of older adults compared two types of workouts to see if either type lowered inflammation (Kohut *et al.*, 2006). In this study, 83 adults, ages 64 to 87, were randomized to either cardio or flexibility/resistance conditions. The cardio workouts were 45 minutes at 60% to 80% of maximal cardiac effort, three times a week for 10 months. The flexibility/resistance workouts were 45 minutes of resistance and flexibility training, three times a week, also for 10 months. Both types of exercise led to improved levels of depression, optimism, and sense of coherence: the three psychological measures the researchers assessed. At the end of 10 months, the cardio workout had the most impact on inflammation. Participants in the cardio condition had significant reductions in C-reactive protein, IL-6, and IL-18. TNF-α levels improved with both the cardio and the flexibility/resistance program. These effects were independent of depression, optimism, or sense of coherence.

Exercise also had a positive effect on wound healing, and this is an indirect measure of systemic inflammation (Emery *et al.*, 2005). In this study, participants were randomized into exercise and control conditions and were then brought into the laboratory and given a punch biopsy. The researchers then monitored participants' rate of wound healing. The average number of days for the wound to heal in the exercise group was 29 days. In the control group, it was 38 days. Exercise one hour a day, three days a week lowered perceived stress and improved wound healing. This study is of interest because we know from this group's other studies that wound healing is impaired when stress or hostility levels are high (e.g., Kiecolt-Glaser *et al.*, 2005). Stress and hostility both increase systemic inflammation. When systemic inflammation is high, wound healing is impaired because proinflammatory cytokines are in the blood stream and not at the wound site where they belong (Kiecolt-Glaser *et al.*, 2005). The Emery *et al.* (2005) study indicates that exercise improves wound healing by lowering levels of circulating systemic cytokines.

Overall level of fitness was also related to inflammation in another recent study (Hamer & Steptoe, 2007). The sample was 207 men and women from London who had no history or symptoms of heart disease and were not being treated for hypertension, inflammatory disease, or allergy. Participants were given two mentally stressful tasks in the laboratory (a computerized Stroop test or mirror tracing task). Researchers drew blood and measured heart rate via a submaximal exercise test. A high-systolic blood pressure indicated a low level of fitness. Participants who responded with higher systolic blood pressure to stress also had a higher IL-6 and TNF-α response. The TNF-α response to stress was five times greater in the low-fitness group compared to the high-fitness group. The authors concluded that participants who were physically fit had a lower inflammation response when under stress. They believed that this was another way that exercise protected individuals from heart disease and other conditions.

Exercise and Breastfeeding

As the above-cited studies indicate, exercise is helpful in lowering systemic inflammation and treating depression. Yet mothers may be concerned that it will negatively impact breastfeeding. Only a few studies have specifically addressed this topic. These studies have generally observed that exercise had no negative effects on breastfeeding. For example, a recent Cochrane Review found that neither diet nor exercise for weight loss appeared to impact breastfeeding adversely (Amorin *et al.*, 2007). However, the authors noted that there was very little research on this topic and that more information was needed before they could say that for certain.

In a qualitative study, six Australian mothers perceived that exercise had reduced their milk supply, although this was not independently confirmed (Rich *et al.*, 2004). These same women reported that exercise reduced their stress, improved weight control and energy, and enhanced the mother-child relationship. Another Australian study (Su *et al.*, 2007) examined the relationship between mothers' exercise, initiation and duration of breastfeeding, and exercise's effect on infant growth. The participants were 587 mothers recruited at birth. Mothers were interviewed seven times over a period of 12 months. At 6 to 12 months, exercise had not decreased breastfeeding duration. At 12 months, exercise had no significant impact on infant growth. This applied to both women who were fully breastfeeding and those who did "any" amount of breastfeeding. The researchers concluded that their study should reassure health care providers that exercise while breastfeeding is safe and important for maintaining health.

Those studies suggest that exercise is generally safe for breastfeeding mothers. A more specific question regarding exercise and breastfeeding has to do with lactic acid. Does exercise cause lactic acid to build up in mothers' milk so that babies won't breastfeed or refuse to take it? A study of 12 lactating women sought to answer this question (Quinn & Carey, 1999). In this study, milk and blood samples were taken after a non-exercise session (control), after maximal exercise, and after a session that was 20% below the maximal range. They found that in women with an adequate maternal caloric intake, moderate exercise did not increase lactic acid in breastmilk nor cause babies to reject it. When women exercised in the "hard" range (using the perceived exertion scale), lactic acid increased. The authors recommended exercise in a moderate range because it neither increases lactic acid accumulation in the breastmilk nor alters babies' willingness to breastfeed.

Summary

In summary, exercise is a highly effective treatment for depression—alone or in combination with other treatments. It appears to have no negative effect on breastfeeding, and it can be a viable alternative treatment if mothers refuse medications.

The one challenge with exercise is getting mothers to do it. When they are depressed, it is probably the last thing they feel like doing. But they may be motivated to try when they realize it's an effective alternative to medications. Blumenthal *et al.* (2007) found a slightly higher remission in the supervised versus at-home exercise groups, likely because compliance rates were higher. A similar approach, perhaps involving a mothers' exercise group, may be useful for mothers who want to give this modality a try. Exercise in a group setting may also provide another useful function—social support, the subject of the next section.

Table 6: Exercise to Achieve an Antidepressant Effect
For mild-to-moderate depression
• **Frequency:** 2 to 3 times a week
• **Intensity:** moderate
• **Duration:** 20 to 30 minutes
For major depression
• **Frequency:** 3 to 5 times a week
• **Intensity:** 60% to 85% maximum capacity
• **Duration:** 45 to 60 minutes

SOCIAL SUPPORT

In a paper on integrative care for women with postpartum depression, LoCicero *et al.* (1997) stated that we must understand women in their social and community contexts if we are to effectively prevent and treat depression. They proposed that communities coordinate a network of services and resources, routinely screen for postpartum depression, and improve provision of perinatal health care. Eleven years later, this is still good advice. We've known for a number of years that social support for mothers is a good idea. Social support is a key factor in preventing depression both during the perinatal period and across the lifespan. Only more recently have we learned that social support has a discernable physical effect—and, indeed, changes the way our brains react to stress. Below is a summary of research on how social support prevents postpartum depression and what happens when women do not have it.

Social Support and Prevention of Depression

Webster and colleagues (2000b) found that women with low social support were significantly more likely to be depressed by 16 weeks postpartum in a prospective, hospital-based study. Women were more vulnerable to depression when they had low support from friends and family, conflict with their partners, and felt their partners did not love them. In another study (Webster *et al.*, 2000a), women with low support during pregnancy reported poorer health during pregnancy and postpartum and were more likely to have postpartum depression. Women without support were more likely to delay seeking prenatal care, but to seek medical care more frequently once they did.

In a study of 191 low-income women, Ritter *et al.* (2000) found that women with good social support were less likely to become depressed. In addition, women with high levels of support also had higher levels of self-esteem. More recently, an Australian study (Haslam *et al.*, 2006) found that women whose parents provided emotional support and who had high self-efficacy had lower levels of postpartum depression. This study included 247 pregnant and postpartum women. Mothers were assessed in their last trimester of pregnancy and at four weeks postpartum. Contrary to prediction, partner support did not influence levels of postpartum depression. The authors hypothesized that support from women's parents likely increased mothers' sense of competence and self-efficacy in caring for their new babies. In addition, support from parents may have been more specific to the needs of new mothers than partner support.

A qualitative study of 41 Canadian mothers found that social support was important for women's recovery from postpartum depression (Letourneau *et al.*, 2007). In this study, mothers identified two types of support that were most helpful in their recovery: instrumental support (e.g., help with household chores) and informational support (e.g., information about postpartum depression). Affirmation support was more helpful when it came from other mothers who could empathize with their experiences, rather than from people who had never been depressed. Mothers also identified partners, friends, family, other mothers, and health care providers as important sources of support. The mothers in this study indicated that they preferred one-on-one to group or telephone support, especially in the beginning. However, once mothers started to recover, they found that group support was helpful.

Efficacy of Community-Based Care

Some studies found that community-based care prevents postpartum depression, but these findings have been mixed. In a study of 2,064 women, half were assigned to midwife care tailored to the women's individual needs. The others were assigned to standard care. At four months postpartum, women in the flexible-care group had significantly better mental health than women in the standard-care group. The authors concluded that midwife-led, flexible care significantly improved new mothers' mental health and reduced the risk of postpartum depression (MacArthur *et al.*, 2002).

A study from England had different results. This study sought to determine whether additional support in the first month postpartum increased maternal health and breastfeeding rates and decreased the risk of postpartum depression (Morrell et al., 2000). There were 623 women in the study. Half were assigned to receive home visits, and the other half received standard care. At six weeks postpartum, there were no significant differences in health status, use of social services, depression, or breastfeeding rates. The mothers were very satisfied with the home visits, however.

A study from South Africa found that home visiting improved mother-infant interaction, but not depression (Cooper et al., 2002). In this study, 64 women were randomly assigned to receive either usual care or home visits by trained community volunteers. The home visitors provided emotional support and taught mothers to be more responsive to their babies, using items from the Neonatal Behavioral Assessment Scale. This intervention had no significant impact on maternal mood (although it was marginally better for mothers in the intervention group), but mothers in the intervention group had significantly more positive emotions when interacting with their babies.

Community-based care even helps in the general population. As described earlier, patient non-compliance with antidepressants can be a substantial problem (Olfson et al., 2006). Fortunately, it can be increased. Simon and colleagues (2000) found that telephone follow-up by a case manager significantly improved patient compliance with antidepressant treatment. Patients with case managers had a 50% improvement in depression and a lower probability of major depression at the six-month follow-up than those who received standard care. The telephone follow-up consisted of a five-minute introductory telephone call and two 10-to-15 minute calls at eight and 16 weeks after the initial prescription. The case managers also communicated with doctors about whether there were side effects or whether the patient might be under-medicated (i.e., still showing moderate levels of depression). The case managers also assisted with arrangements for follow-up visits, but did not provide psychotherapy. This type of community-based followup could potentially be added to any treatment for depression.

Education Support

Educational support is a key component of many community-based programs designed to reduce the risk of depression. The results of these programs, however, have also been mixed. In one education program (Elliot et al., 2000), women identified during pregnancy as being at-risk for depression were randomly assigned to a preventive intervention or a control group.

At three months postpartum, 19% of the women in the "Preparation for Parenthood" group were depressed compared with 39% of the mothers who received standard care. These findings were true only for first-time mothers.

Another study found that education during pregnancy was not helpful in reducing postpartum depression (Hayes *et al.*, 2001). In this study, women were randomly assigned to either an education condition or normal care. Depression was assessed during pregnancy and at two points postpartum. There were no differences between the control and intervention groups and no relevant influence of social support or demographic variables. There was an improvement in depressive symptoms for both groups over time: both were more likely to be depressed during pregnancy than at either point postpartum. The authors concluded that their findings challenge two strongly held beliefs by professionals in the perinatal health field. First, that depression can be reduced through education. And second, that interventions done during pregnancy can endure into the postpartum period.

In summary, social support is a useful modality in preventing and possibly treating postpartum depression. The studies summarized above indicate that a wide range of support is helpful: emotional, instrumental, informational, and affirmational. While support did not always improve rates of depression, it raised self-esteem and self-efficacy and improved mothers' interactions with their babies. Some of the most intriguing research in this field has examined the impact of social support on health, and this research suggests a possible mechanism by which support lowers risk for depression.

The Health-Enhancing Effects of Social Support

Intriguingly, it appears that social support, always known as helpful for preventing depression, also has a physiological effect. Much of this research comes from the cardiology, health psychology, and psychocardiology literature. These fields have identified low social support, low social integration, or perceived low social status as being risk factors for heart disease. Given the strong link between depression and heart disease, social support may indeed provide insight into possible mechanisms by which lack of support increases risk for depression (Kendall-Tackett, 2007b).

Many of the studies on this topic have examined the health effects of marriage, which seems particularly protective of men's health. In a review of the literature on marriage and health, Kiecolt-Glaser and Newton (2001) found that being married reduced premature mortality by 500% for men. For women, marriage reduced premature mortality by only 50%—likely because women have larger social networks outside of marriage than men.

In data from the Framingham Offspring Study, married men were half as likely to die during the follow-up period as unmarried men (Eaker *et al.*, 2007). The Framingham Offspring Study is the second-generation of data collection from the Framingham Heart Study, a major study of cardiovascular disease, now following the second and third generations of study participants. The results were a bit more complex for women. Marital status alone was not enough to prolong life; however, aspects of how women handled marital conflict were. Women who "self-silenced" in conflicts were four times more likely to die compared with those who did not. The findings were true even after adjusting for systolic blood pressure, age, body mass index, cigarette smoking, diabetes, and cholesterol.

While the effects of marriage on health are generally good, ongoing marital strife is not. In fact, it increases the risk of heart disease, particularly for women. A 13-year longitudinal study of married women found that women with poor-quality marriages had higher rates of several markers for cardiovascular disease: low HDL cholesterol, high triglycerides, and higher body mass index, blood pressure, depression, and anger (Gallo *et al.*, 2003). In a study from Sweden, Orth-Gomer and colleagues (2000) followed 292 women for five years after a myocardial infarction. They found that women with high levels of marital strife were nearly three times more likely to have another heart attack or other coronary event, than women who were married, but not distressed. This relationship held even after adjusting for age, estrogen levels, education, and smoking.

One way that relationships may increase cardiovascular risk is by impacting sleep. Two recent studies have examined the relationship between security of adult attachments and sleep quality. Sleep is a physiologically vulnerable state. In order to sleep soundly, people must feel sufficiently secure, so they can downregulate vigilance and alertness. To do so, one must be secure in social relationships (Troxel *et al.*, 2007).

In the first study, 78 married adults completed questionnaires about their sleep quality, quality of current partnership (secure versus insecure attachment), and depression (Carmichael & Reis, 2005). The sleep questionnaire asked about seven aspects of sleep, including perceived sleep quality, sleep latency (time to get to sleep), sleep duration, habitual sleep efficiency, sleep disturbances, and use of sleep medications. Using structural equation modeling, the researchers found that married participants who were anxious about their current relationships reported poorer sleep quality, even after controlling for depression. Women with insecure attachments were concerned that their partners were emotionally unavailable and not trustworthy. The researchers indicated that one limitation to their study was that they used a self-report measure of sleep, rather than assessing sleep directly.

Troxel and colleagues (2007) addressed that limitation by using polysomnographic studies to assess sleep directly. In a study of 107 women with recurrent major depression, marital status and security of that relationship predicted quality and efficiency of sleep. If women had anxious attachments, particularly if they were separated or widowed, they had a significantly smaller percentage of stage 3-4 sleep than women who were currently partnered and had secure attachments. The authors noted the importance of stage 3-4 sleep in protecting individuals from cardiovascular and metabolic diseases.

McEwen (2003) reported that even short periods of sleep deprivation can elevate cortisol and glucose levels and can increase both insulin and insulin resistance. Sleep deprivation also provokes an inflammatory response since the body thinks it's under attack. Long-term sleep deprivation can seriously impair health, and this could be a health risk factor for women who are not in stable, secure relationships.

One intriguing question relevant to postpartum women is whether there are similar effects when women sleep near versus away from their babies. What is the impact on sleep when women are separated from their babies at night? Do they also enter a state of hypervigilance? Does this increase the inflammatory response because it impacts sleep quality? Do women who sleep near their babies have a higher percentage of stage 3-4 sleep? These are questions to explore in future studies, with important implications for how we counsel mothers.

When Support is Absent: Social Isolation and Cardiac Risk factors

Much of what we know about the health effects of social support comes from studying its absence—social isolation and an inability to trust others. This psychological state also triggers the inflammatory response. Individuals who expect the worst from people become hypervigilant to rejection in social relationships. This world view has discernable, physical sequelae.

A study of 6,814 healthy men and women found that participants with higher levels of cynical distrust, chronic stress, or depression had higher levels of inflammation (Ranjit *et al.*, 2007). Indicators of inflammation included elevated C-reactive protein, IL-6, and fibrinogen. Chronic stress was associated with higher IL-6 and C-reactive protein, and depression was associated with higher IL-6. All are risk factors for heart disease.

In elderly men, low social integration was associated with increased fibrinogen (Loucks *et al.*, 2005). The researchers calculated social integration using marital status, number of contacts with family and friends, frequency of religious service attendance, and participation in volunteer organizations. Fibrinogen is a soluble protein that aids in clotting. Because it increases the speed of platelet aggregation and thrombus formation, a high level of fibrinogen is a risk factor for cardiovascular disease.

In a sample of middle-aged and older adults, social isolation increased levels of another cardiac risk factor: coronary artery calcification. Being single or widowed was related to calcification, whereas health behaviors, socioeconomic status, and depression were not (Kop *et al.*, 2005). This relationship remained even after controlling for other cardiac risk factors.

Perceived Social Status and Cardiovascular Risk

Where you fall on the social hierarchy also has an impact on your cardiovascular health. If a woman perceives that she has low social status—because of education, ethnicity, vocation, or income level—it raises the risk of cardiovascular disease via several physiological mechanisms. Low social status was associated with low-grade inflammation in a sample of 121 White and African American men and women (Hong *et al.*, 2006). In this sample, researchers measured soluble intercellular adhesion molecule (sICAM) and endothelin-1 (ET-1). Both are measures of vascular inflammation. Men and women in the lowest social class had the highest levels of sICAM and ET-1. Low status was also reflected in the measure of C-reactive protein in another study of middle-aged and older adults (McDade *et al.*, 2006). In this sample, African Americans, women, and those with lower education had the highest levels of CRP. However, ethnic group differences disappeared once health behaviors were factored in. The authors concluded that psychosocial stress and health behaviors are both important determinants of systemic inflammation and increased cardiac risk.

Low parental education level, another marker of social status, predicted metabolic and cardiovascular risk factors in Black and White high school students. Low-status students had higher insulin levels, higher glucose, greater insulin resistance, higher LDL and lower HDL cholesterol, higher waist circumference, and higher body mass index than high-status students (Goodman *et al.*, 2005). Socioeconomic status was also associated with higher basal cortisol levels and catecholamines in a sample of 193 Black and White adults (Cohen *et al.*, 2006). Finally, perceived discrimination was related to coronary artery calcification in middle-aged African American women (Lewis *et al.*, 2006).

How supported you feel in your neighborhood also influences your health. Adverse neighborhoods can compound the negative health impact of people living with chronic stress. In one study of this effect, 147 caregivers of patients with Alzheimer's disease were compared with 147 non-caregivers on three measures of neighborhood characteristics (Brummett *et al.*, 2005). An adverse neighborhood was one where there was high crime and where neighbors were hostile or indifferent to each other. Sample items asked subjects if they had "untrustworthy neighbors" or if "people insult or bother others." Neighborhood characteristics did compound the chronic stress of caregiving. Specifically, caregivers living in high-crime, low-trust neighborhoods had impaired glucose control, measured by fasting plasma glucose and glycosylated hemoglobin concentration (the standard marker for measurement of average plasma glucose). These findings were true even after controlling for age, race, gender, relation to care recipient, body mass index, income, and education.

Summary

While the research on cardiac risk factors may not seem immediately relevant to postpartum depression, it demonstrates that our social relationships either increase or decrease our vulnerability to stress. This vulnerability manifests through several physiological mechanisms, including inflammation. What these findings indicate is that humans are social animals and that social support, social integration, and perceived social status have measurable effects on health. Indeed, loved ones and others in our social orbit help regulate our internal states. What is particularly interesting about these findings is their continuity throughout the lifespan, from infancy to old age. In studies of term infants, separation from mother causes perturbations to both heart rate and

Table 7: Social Support for New Mothers
• Social support is critical for the prevention and treatment of postpartum depression.
• Support can take several forms: informational, emotional, instrumental, and affirmational.
• It can be offered to mothers one-on-one or in group settings. Mothers' preference and need can vary by type of support offered and where a mother is in her recovery.
• Lack of support has physiological consequences, including increased inflammation, which increases women's vulnerability to depression.

glucose levels (Christensson *et al.*, 1992). During adulthood, disruptions to social networks result in the end-state diseases related to disturbances in heart rate and glucose levels: heart disease, metabolic syndrome, and diabetes. With regard to new mothers, these findings suggest that social support is critical for new mothers–for both their physical and mental health. These findings also contradict commonly given advice that may separate mothers and babies. This separation may trigger a stress response in mothers and be counterproductive to their recovery. Instead of separating them, an alternative is to support mother and baby together. This would suppress the stress response and allow mothers to gradually grow into their new role. A summary of social support for new mothers is listed on **Table 7**.

In closing, Lewis, Amini, and Lannon (2000) noted the importance of our relationships in maintaining our physical and mental health, and observed the following:

> Adults remain social animals; they continue to require a source of stabilization outside themselves. That open-loop design means that in some important ways, people cannot be stable on their own—not should or shouldn't be, but can't be (p. 86, emphasis added).

PSYCHOTHERAPY

Mothers can experience social support through informal networks of friends and family, or, they can experience support through more formal channels, such as psychotherapy. As described in an earlier section, psychotherapy is a frontline therapy for postpartum depression. In clinical trials, psychotherapy has proven as effective as medications, with lower rates of relapse (Rupke *et al.*, 2006). Researchers have studied two types of psychotherapy with regard to depression in new mothers: cognitive-behavioral therapy and interpersonal psychotherapy. These are described below.

Cognitive-Behavioral Therapy

Cognitive-behavioral therapy is a highly effective form of psychotherapy. In numerous clinical trials, cognitive-behavioral therapy has proven to be as powerful as medications for treating depression, anxiety, chronic pain, and obsessive compulsive disorder. Moreover, patients who received cognitive therapy did better on follow-up, were less likely to relapse, and were less likely to drop out of treatment than those who received medications alone (Antonuccio *et al.*, 1995; Rupke *et al.*, 2006).

Cognitive therapy is based on the premise that distortions in thinking cause depression. Some examples of cognitive distortions include that a negative situation will never change, that it encompasses many areas of a woman's life, and that when negative things happen, it is because of some character flaw or defect in the person. Cognitive therapy teaches patients to recognize and counter these thoughts (Rupke *et al.*, 2006). The goal is to help patients identify distorted beliefs and replace them with more rational ones. For example, is it really true that there is "nothing" you can do to change a situation?

Cognitive therapy is not simply learning to think "happy" thoughts, nor is it mere "talk therapy." Cognitive therapy can change the brain. Two studies compared cognitive therapy to medications on two serotonergic conditions: obsessive-compulsive disorder (Baxter *et al.*, 1992) and panic disorder (Prasko *et al.*, 2004). In both studies, the outcome variable was change in positron emission tomography (PET) scans of the brain before and after treatment. Before therapy, both groups showed abnormalities in brain metabolism. After treatment, both groups had improved PET scans, but there was no difference between the groups. In other words, cognitive therapy caused the same changes in the brain that medications had in both studies.

Cognitive therapy has also been used to treat postpartum depression in several studies. In a study from England, 87 women with postpartum depression were randomized to one of four conditions: fluoxetine or placebo, plus one or six sessions of cognitive-behavioral therapy (Appleby *et al.*, 1997). Health visitors who attended a brief training provided the therapy. The sessions were designed to offer reassurance and advice on topics of specific concern to new mothers. The initial session was one hour, and subsequent sessions were 30 minutes each. Four weeks after treatment, all four groups had improved. Not surprisingly, women receiving fluoxetine improved significantly more than women receiving the placebo, and women receiving six sessions of counseling improved significantly more than women who only received one session. There was no advantage to women receiving both medication and counseling beyond the first session. Cognitive-behavioral therapy was as effective as medication.

In another study (Misri et al., 2004), researchers added cognitive therapy to medications for moderate-to-severe postpartum depression. In this study, depressed, anxious mothers were assigned to receive paroxetine alone or paroxetine with cognitive-group therapy. Mothers in both groups improved after treatment, and there was no significant difference between the groups. From these results, there appeared to be no additional benefit of adding cognitive therapy to medications. A study from Australia compared standard care, group cognitive therapy, or individual counseling for women with postpartum depression. After 12 weeks, both types of psychological treatment were superior to standard care, and the researchers concluded that individual counseling was as effective as group cognitive therapy (Milgrom et al., 2005).

Cognitive therapy was not effective in preventing depression in mothers of very preterm babies, however (Hagan et al., 2004). In this study, 101 mothers of very preterm babies received six sessions of cognitive therapy. They were compared with 98 mothers who received standard care. There were no differences in onset or duration of depression between the two groups, and 37% of mothers were depressed. The authors indicated that mothers of very preterm infants had high rates of stress and depression, and that a six-week intervention did not alter the prevalence of depression in this group.

A study from Glasgow with a non-postpartum sample combined cognitive therapy with mindfulness meditation in an eight-week course for people with relapsing, recurring depression (Finucane & Mercer, 2006). With a sample of 13 patients, the mean pre-course depression score was 35.7. After the course, it was 17.8. Anxiety had a similar decline. Mindfulness was added to address the ruminative thinking style that increases vulnerability to relapsing depression. Ruminative thinking involves rehashing personal shortcomings and problematic situations. This style of thinking perpetuates rather than relieves stress. Mindfulness teaches patients to let go of negative thinking and to be open to what is there without aversion or attachment. Patients in this trial found the addition of mindfulness helpful in preventing subsequent episodes of depression.

In summary, what we think and how we frame the world has a substantial impact on our mental health. Cognitive therapy is a powerful way to treat even major depression. Not only does it treat depression, it can also produce measurable changes in the brain that are comparable to those produced by antidepressants. It also has no impact on breastfeeding and is a viable, effective alternative treatment.

Interpersonal Psychotherapy

Interpersonal psychotherapy is a newer type of psychotherapy that has also proven effective in the treatment of depression. In a recent NIMH-collaborative research study, interpersonal psychotherapy was as effective as tricyclic antidepressants and cognitive therapy, and was effective for almost 70% of the patients (Tolman, 2001).

Interpersonal psychotherapy is based on attachment theory and the interpersonal theories of Harry Stack Sullivan. Disturbances in the key relationships are hypothesized as being responsible for depression (Stuart & O'Hara, 1995). Interpersonal psychotherapy addresses four problem areas: role transitions, interpersonal disputes, grief, and interpersonal deficits. On a client's first visit, a specific problem is identified, and the client and therapist begin work on that issue. Mothers complete an interpersonal inventory and review information about key relationships, the nature of current communications, and how having a baby has changed those relationships (Grigoriadis & Ravitz, 2007). The key difference between interpersonal psychotherapy and other types is its focus. Interpersonal psychotherapy specifically targets improving a woman's relationships and discussing her role transitions. Because its focus is more specific than a more diffuse supportive psychotherapy, it can be delivered in fewer sessions, and preliminary evidence suggests that it is more effective.

With postpartum women, the goal of interpersonal psychotherapy is to help them with role transitions and changes in roles they have already established (Stuart & O'Hara, 1995). A related goal is to assist women in building or making better use of existing support (Grigoriadis & Ravitz, 2007). In a study of 120 women with postpartum major depression (O'Hara *et al.*, 2000), women were assigned to either interpersonal psychotherapy or wait-list conditions for 12 weeks. The therapists were trained in interpersonal psychotherapy, and they followed a standardized treatment manual. O'Hara *et al.* found that women in the therapy group had significantly lower depression scores than women in the wait-list group at four, eight, and 12 weeks after treatment. The rate of recovery from depression was also significantly higher for women in the therapy group, and they scored better on postpartum adjustment and social support. The authors noted that interpersonal therapy was effective for women with postpartum depression. It reduced depressive symptoms and improved social adjustment. The authors felt that interpersonal psychotherapy represents a viable alternative to pharmacotherapy, especially for women who are breastfeeding.

Klier, Muzik, Rosenbaum, and Lenz (2001) also found interpersonal psychotherapy effective for 17 women with postpartum depression. In this study, interpersonal psychotherapy was used in group therapy. Women had significantly decreased depression after attending the group, and this was still true at the six-month follow-up. The authors noted some limitations in their study, such as small sample size, lack of a control group, and possible bias in the therapist's assessment of the women. Reay and colleagues (2006) had similar findings in their preliminary study of 18 mothers with postpartum depression. In this study, mothers participated in a program of interpersonal psychotherapy with two individual sessions and eight group sessions. Mothers' depression decreased significantly after treatment. However, 67% of the mothers were also on antidepressants, and there was no control group.

Another study compared interpersonal psychotherapy to parenting education for 50 low-income, pregnant women with major depression (Spinelli & Endicott, 2003). Both interpersonal psychotherapy and the control education condition were administered over 16 weeks. Women in their sample had a number of severe risk factors for depression: 47% had a history of childhood abuse (28% sexual abuse, 25% physical abuse, 6% both) and 73% had a history of major depression. In addition, many had chaotic home environments, unstable relationships, or partners involved in criminal activity. At the end of 16 weeks, significantly more women in the treatment group had a greater than 50% reduction in depressive symptoms on the Hamilton Depression Scale and the Beck Depression Inventory. The authors concluded that interpersonal psychotherapy was an effective treatment for depression during pregnancy and should be a first-line treatment.

Interpersonal psychotherapy has also proven helpful in preventing postpartum depression in high-risk women (Zlotnick *et al.*, 2006). In this study, 99 low-income pregnant women were randomly assigned to receive standard antenatal care or standard care plus an intervention based on interpersonal therapy. The goal of the intervention was to improve women's close, personal relationships, change their expectations about these relationships, build their social networks, and help them master their transition to motherhood. The intervention was four 60-minute sessions during pregnancy, with one "booster" session after delivery. The intervention was delivered in a group setting. At three months postpartum, 4% of the intervention group became depressed compared to 20% of the control group.

Interpersonal psychotherapy was used to treat low-income, depressed adolescents in five school-based mental health clinics in New York City (Mufson *et al.*, 2004). In this study, 63 teens with depression or dysthymia were randomly assigned to receive 16 weeks of interpersonal psychotherapy or 16 weeks of treatment as usual. "Treatment as usual" included whatever individual psychotherapy the teens would have received if the program were not in place. The sample was 84% female and 71% Hispanic. By the end of the intervention, teens receiving interpersonal therapy had significantly fewer depressive symptoms, had better social functioning, greater clinical improvement, and a greater decrease in clinical severity on the Clinical Global Impressions scale. The authors noted that the largest treatment effects occurred for the older and more severely depressed adolescents. They also noted that although medications are often seen as frontline treatment for depressed teens, these were difficult to access through school clinics. Moreover, minority families were reluctant to accept antidepressants. Of the four teens in the study that were prescribed antidepressants, all had poor compliance with their treatment regimens. The authors concluded that this school-based program was a viable alternative to medications for depressed, low-income adolescents.

In addition to data from clinical trials, two recent literature reviews indicated that interpersonal psychotherapy is effective and well-suited to the treatment of postpartum depression. In their review of four clinical trials, Weissman (2007) found that women who received 12 to 16 weeks of interpersonal psychotherapy showed a significant reduction of symptoms compared with women who received standard care. Weissman also indicated that interpersonal psychotherapy can be provided by mental health professionals, health care providers, or trained laypeople. Grigoridadis and

Ravitz (2007) also concluded that interpersonal psychotherapy is an effective treatment for postpartum depression. They indicated that this approach can be easily integrated into primary care settings, and that it is short-term, highly effective, and ideally suited to the needs of postpartum women.

Anti-inflammatory Effects of Psychotherapy

Although evidence is quite preliminary, both cognitive therapy and interpersonal psychotherapy likely have an anti-inflammatory effect. Interpersonal psychotherapy's effect is due to increasing the amount and quality of support, which was described in the previous section.

Some of the more interesting findings are regarding the physiological effect of what we think. Of particular relevance is the research on the health effects of hostility. Hostility is of interest because it is a particular way of looking at the world. People high in hostility tend to attribute negative motives to others, and have difficulty trusting others and establishing close relationships. It also likely increases inflammation. In one study, hostility was associated with higher levels of circulating proinflammatory cytokines (IL-1α, IL-1β, and IL-8) in 44 healthy, non-smoking, premenopausal women. The combination of depression and hostility led to the highest levels of IL-1β, IL-8, and TNF-α (Suarez et al., 2004). There was a dose-response effect: the more severe the depression and hostility, the greater the production of cytokines.

More recently, Suarez (2006) studied 135 healthy patients (75 men, 60 women), with no symptoms of diabetes. He found that women with higher levels of depression and hostility had higher levels of fasting insulin, glucose, and insulin resistance. These findings were not true for men, and they were independent of other risk factors for metabolic syndrome, including body mass index, age, fasting triglycerides, exercise regularity, or ethnicity. These findings were significant since pre-study glucose levels were in the non-diabetic range. The author noted that inflammation, as indicated by elevated plasma levels of IL-6 and C-reactive protein, may mediate the relationship between depression and hostility and risk of type 2 diabetes and cardiovascular disease, possibly because they increase insulin resistance.

In another recent study, Kiecolt-Glaser et al. (2005) found that couples who were high in hostility had higher levels of circulating proinflammatory cytokines. As a result, the rate of wound healing for the high-hostility couples was 60% slower than for low-hostility couples. High-hostility couples had fewer cytokines at the wound site, where they were supposed to be, and high levels circulating systemically, where they were more likely to impair health and increase the risk of age-related diseases.

Cognitive therapy specifically addresses beliefs like hostility. Since negative cognitions increase inflammation, we could predict that reducing their occurrence would lower inflammation. That is indeed what Doering and colleagues (2007) found in their study of women after coronary bypass surgery. They found that clinically depressed women had a higher incidence of in-hospital fevers and infections in the six months after surgery due, in part, to decreases in natural killer cell cytotoxicity. An 8-week program of cognitive-behavioral therapy reduced depression, improved natural killer cell cytotoxicity, and decreased IL-6 and C-reactive protein. Because the immune system was functioning more effectively, this intervention decreased postoperative infectious diseases.

In summary, the two types of psychotherapy reviewed in this section likely decrease inflammation, but through different mechanisms. Interpersonal psychotherapy focuses on improving social support, which downregulates the inflammatory response. Cognitive therapy lowers inflammation by changing the negative beliefs that upregulate stress and inflammatory response. What both forms of psychotherapy have in common is that they affect both physical and emotional health.

Summary of Psychotherapy

Cognitive therapy and interpersonal therapy are both effective treatments for postpartum depression. At this time, there is more empirical support for cognitive therapy, and mothers may have an easier time locating a practitioner who can provide it. But interpersonal psychotherapy shows great promise for both preventing and treating postpartum depression. Indeed, at some point in the future, interpersonal psychotherapy may supplant cognitive therapy as the frontline psychotherapy for postpartum depression. Additional information on psychotherapy is found in **Table 8.**

Table 8: Resources on Psychotherapy
Cognitive Therapy
The National Association of Cognitive-Behavioral Therapists
http://www.nacbt.org
Association of Behavioral and Cognitive Therapies (ABCT)
http://www.aabt.org
Interpersonal Psychotherapy
International Society for Interpersonal Psychotherapy
http://www.interpersonalpsychotherapy.org/
General Resources
National Alliance on Mental Illness
http://www.nami.org
To locate a therapist
http://www.therapistlocator.net

ST. JOHN'S WORT

The final treatment modality is St. John's wort (Hypericum perforatum): the most widely used herbal antidepressant in the world (Dugoua *et al.*, 2006). Herbalists have used St. John's wort since the Middle Ages. At that time, it was used to treat insanity resulting from "attacks of the devil." It derives its name from St. John's Day (June 24) because it blooms near this day on the medieval church calendar. "Wort" is the old English word for a medicinal plant. It is native to Great Britain, Wales, and northern Europe. Since settlers brought it to North America in the 1700s (Balch, 2002; Humphrey, 2003), it is now a common wildflower in the northeastern and north central U.S.

Efficacy of St. John's Wort

A large body of evidence indicates that St. John's wort effectively treats depression (Sarris, 2007; Werneke *et al.*, 2006). Most of the earlier research has been done in Germany, where St. John's wort is widely used and, indeed, is the preferred treatment for depression. Standard antidepressants are tried only after St. John's wort has failed (Linde *et al.*, 1996; Wurglies & Schubert-Zsilavecz, 2006). Evidence for St. John's wort's effectiveness can be found in both review articles and in results of randomized clinical trials.

Review Articles

In a meta-analysis of 23 randomized trials, Linde and colleagues (1996) found that hypericum extracts were superior to placebos and were as effective as antidepressants in treating depression. Patients taking St. John's wort were less likely to drop out of studies and reported fewer side effects than their counterparts taking antidepressants. Placebo groups (across 13 studies) had an average response rate of 22.3%, compared with 55% of the hypericum groups.

A review of 22 studies (Whiskey *et al.*, 2001) and another with 27 trials (Lawvere & Mahoney, 2005) had similar findings. The authors of both reviews found that St. John's wort was more effective than a placebo and as effective as antidepressants. They also concluded that side effects were more common with antidepressants than with St. John's wort. A final review indicated that there was "very strong evidence" of St. John's wort's effectiveness for mild-to-moderate depression (Duguoa *et al.*, 2006).

Data from Clinical Trials

A number of clinical trials have compared the efficacy of various St. John's wort extracts to either a placebo or an antidepressant. In one trial (Lecrubier *et al.*, 2002), 375 patients were randomized to receive either St. John's wort (Hypericum perforatum Extract WS 5570) or a placebo for six weeks to treat mild-to-moderate depression. At the end of six weeks, patients receiving St. John's wort had significantly lower scores on the Hamilton Depression Rating Scale. Significantly more patients were in remission or had a response to treatment than patients receiving the placebo. Both groups had similar rates of adverse effects. Fifty-three percent of the patients in the St. John's wort group responded to treatment, compared with 42% of the placebo group. The authors concluded that St. John's wort was safe and effective for the treatment of mild-to-moderate depression.

Two randomized trials compared St. John's wort to the tricyclic antidepressant imipramine. The first randomized trial compared St. John's wort (Hypericum extract ZE 117) to imipramine for 324 outpatients with mild-to-moderate depression (Woelk, 2000). After six weeks of treatment, St. John's wort was as effective as imipramine in lowering depressive symptoms. However, adverse effects were significantly more likely in the imipramine group, with 63% reporting adverse effects, but only 39% reporting adverse effects in the St. John's wort group. In addition, only 3% in the St. John's wort group dropped out of the study due to adverse effects versus 16% of the imipramine group. The author concluded that St. John's wort is therapeutically equivalent to imipramine, but it is better tolerated by patients.

The second trial compared St. John's wort (Hypericum extract STEI 300) to a placebo and imipramine. The subjects were 263 primary-care patients with moderate depression. The authors found that St. John's wort was as effective as imipramine for moderately depressed patients after four, six, and eight weeks of treatment (Philipp *et al.*, 1999). Patients in this trial also tolerated St. John's wort better.

Two clinical trials compared St. John's wort to sertraline for major depression. One study had wide press coverage, but unfortunately much of it was misleading (Hypericum Depression Trial Study Group, 2002). In this study, 340 adults with major depression were randomly assigned to receive H Perforatum, a placebo, or sertraline for eight weeks. Subjects responding to the medication could opt to receive still-blinded treatment for another 18 weeks. Depression was assessed at baseline and again at eight weeks. The researchers found no significant difference in depression levels or rate of response between the placebo and St. John's wort. That much was widely reported. What the media did not report was that the same was true for sertraline. The rate of full response was almost identical for the St. John's wort and sertraline groups (24% vs. 25%). The low response rates for both medications suggest limitations to the study. Eight weeks may not have been sufficient for patients with severe depression to recover, or the dosages may have been too low. The authors noted that their findings were not unusual in that approximately 35% of studies of standard antidepressants show no greater efficacy than the placebo.

Another study that same year of patients with major depression had opposite findings. This study (van Gurp *et al.*, 2002) included 87 patients with major depression recruited from Canadian family practice physicians. Patients were randomly assigned to receive either St. John's wort or sertraline. At the end of the 12-week trial, both groups improved, and there was no difference between the two groups. But there were significantly more side effects in the sertraline group at two and four weeks. The authors concluded that St. John's wort, because of its effectiveness and benign side effects, was a good first choice for a primary-care population.

St. John's wort was also compared to paroxetine in a study of 251 patients with acute, moderate-to-severe major depression (Szegedi *et al.*, 2005). In this study, patients were randomly assigned to receive 20 mg paroxetine or 900 mg

St. John's wort (Hypericum extract WS 5570). After two weeks, dosages for non-responders were doubled: 1,800 mg St. John's wort or 40 mg paroxetine. After six weeks of treatment, the response rates were 70% for St. John's wort and 60% for paroxetine. The remission rates for St. John's wort were 50% versus 35% for paroxetine. The authors concluded that St. John's wort was as effective as paroxetine and better tolerated.

Anghelescu and colleagues (2006) also compared the efficacy and safety of Hypericum extract WS 5570 to paroxetine for patients with moderate-to-severe depression. The acute phase of treatment lasted for six weeks, with another four months of follow-up to prevent relapse. The patients improved on both treatments, with no significant difference in efficacy between paroxetine and St. John's wort. The authors noted that St. John's wort was an important alternative to standard antidepressants for depressed patients.

Mechanism for Efficacy

Researchers still do not understand the exact mechanism for St. John's wort's antidepressant effect. Linde *et al.* (1996) noted that hypericum extracts have at least 10 constituents that likely cause its pharmacological effects. St. John's wort is standardized by percentage of hypericin, one of the active constituents. Hypericin was once considered the primary antidepressant component. Researchers no longer believe that this is true (Bratman & Girman, 2003). More recently, researchers have recognized hyperforin as the possible antidepressant constituent (Lawvere & Mahoney, 2005; Muller, 2003; Wurglies & Schubert-Zsilavecz, 2006; Zanoli, 2004). Hyperforin appears to inhibit the reuptake of the monoamines and GABAergic activity (Kuhn & Winston, 2000; Werneke *et al.*, 2006). It may relieve depression by preventing the reuptake of serotonin, the same mechanism as the selective serotonin reuptake inhibitors (SSRIs, e.g., fluoxetine, sertraline). Indeed, Muller (2003) noted that only hyperforin (and its structural analogue, adhyperforin) inhibit neurotransmitter re-uptake.

St. John's wort, and particularly hyperforin, also appears to be anti-inflammatory (Balch, 2002; Dell'Aica *et al.*, 2007; Kuhn & Winston, 2000; Wurglies & Schubert-Zsilavecz, 2006). It also modulates cytokine production (Werneke *et al.*, 2006). Hyperforin has anti-nociceptive (anti-pain) and anti-inflammatory effects in animal studies (Abdel-Salam, 2005). It inhibits the expression of another inflammatory marker—intercellular adhesion molecule

Table 9: Dosage and Safety Information on St. John's wort
Dosage: 300 mg, three times a day
Standardized to: 0.3% hypericin or 2% to 4% hyperforin
Where to Go for Information on Herbs and Herb Safety
www.ConsumerLab.com (rates quality of nutritional products through independent testing)
Institute for Natural Products Research: www.naturalproducts.org/ Humphrey, S. (2003) Nursing mothers' herbal. Minneapolis: Fairview Press.
Herbs for Health magazine: www.discoverherbs.com The Complete German Commission E Monographs available online and for purchase from the American Botanical Council, www.herbalgram.org
National Center for Complementary and Alternative Medicine (NCCAM) http://nccam.nih.gov/health/stjohnswort/sjwataglance.htm
Mayo Clinic St. John's Wort Patient Sheet http://www.mayoclinic.com/ health/st-johns-wort/NS_patient-stjohnswort

(Zhou *et al.*, 2004). In vitro effects show that St. John's wort is anti-oxidant, anti-cyclooxygenase-1, and anti-carcinogenic (Zanoli, 2004).

Only recently has St. John's wort been shown to specifically lower levels of the proinflammatory cytokines involved in depression—and it was not in a study of depression (Hu *et al.*, 2006). The study used an animal model to test whether St. John's wort could counter the toxic side effects of chemotherapy. The investigators specifically investigated whether St. John's wort had an impact on the levels of proinflammatory cytokines, including IL-1β, IL-2, IL-6, IFN-γ, and TNF-α. They found that St. John's wort did protect rats receiving chemotherapy by inhibiting proinflammatory cytokines and intestinal epithelium apoptosis. Although not a study of depression, it was the first to demonstrate that St. John's wort inhibits the cytokines that are high in depression.

Dosage

The dosage of St. John's wort is 900 mg per day (300 mg/three times per day), standardized to 0.3% hypericin and/or 2% to 4% hyperforin (Lawvere

Table 10: Standards for Herbal Preparations
Statement of % standardization of the extract
Statement describing which compounds are standardized
Statement describing which parts of the plant are used in the formulation
Extract ratio (the ratio of extract concentration to crude plant materials, e.g., 1:4)
Recommended daily dosage
Weight and number of capsules or tablets per package
Substantiated structure/function claims
Product expiration date to confirm freshness
A toll-free number and/or Website address for company information and contact
USP: Notation that the manufacturer followed standards of the U.S. Pharmacopeia.
Source: Institute for Natural Products Research (2000).

& Mahoney, 2005). It generally takes four to six weeks to take effect (Bratman & Girman, 2003; Ernst, 2002; Kuhn & Winston, 2000). Dosage information is summarized in **Table 9**.

St. John's wort reaches peak level in the plasma in five hours, with a half-life of 24 to 48 hours. Herbalists often combine it with other herbs to address the range of symptoms that depressed people have. Some of these herbs include lemon balm, kava, schisandra, rosemary, black cohosh, and lavender (Humphrey, 2007; Kuhn & Winston, 2000).

Unfortunately, it can be challenging for women to know if a brand of herbs they purchase is of good quality. As of this writing, the U.S. Pharmacopeia does not verify brands of St. John's wort, but a USP monograph on St. John's wort is due out in 2008. However, ConsumerLabs.com does rate brands of herbs. For a small subscription fee, women can access this resource. There is also information that consumers can look for on supplement labels that give some indication of quality. This information is listed in **Table 10**.

Safety Concerns

Taken by itself, St. John's wort has an excellent safety record, with a very low frequency of adverse reactions (Ernst, 2002; Humphrey, 2003; Muller, 2003). Approximately 2.4% of patients who take St. John's wort develop side effects. The most common are mild stomach discomfort, allergic reactions,

Table 11: Cautions about Drug Interactions with St. John's Wort
St. John's wort affects the way the body processes or breaks down many drugs; in some cases, it may speed or slow a drug's breakdown. Drugs that can be affected include: • Indinavir and possibly other drugs used to control HIV infection • Irinotecan and possibly other drugs used to treat cancer • Cyclosporine, which prevents the body from rejecting transplanted organs • Digoxin, which strengthens heart muscle contractions • Warfarin and related anticoagulants • Birth control pills • Antidepressants
Source: National Center for Complementary & Alternative Medicine (http://nccam.nih.gov/health/stjohnswort/sjwataglance.htm)

skin rashes, tiredness, and restlessness. Like other antidepressants, St. John's wort can trigger an episode of mania in vulnerable patients or patients with bipolar disorder (Bratman & Girman, 2003). St. John's wort can also cause photosensitivity. A review of 38 controlled clinical trials and two meta-analyses on St. John's wort found its safety and side-effect profile to be better than standard antidepressants. The incidence of adverse events ranged from 0% to 6%, which is 10 times less than adverse effects associated with antidepressants (Schultz, 2006).

More concerning is that St. John's wort interacts with several classes of medications and accelerates the metabolism of anticonvulsants, cyclosporins, birth control pills, and others, leading to lower serum levels of the medication than prescribed (Duguoa et al., 2006; Ernst, 2002; Hale, 2006). It can also interact with prescription antidepressants, causing a potentially fatal episode of serotonin syndrome (Bratman & Girman, 2003; Looper, 2007; Werneke et al., 2006). Prescription antidepressants should not be taken while taking St. John's wort (Harkness & Bratman, 2003). Any mothers who are taking St. John's wort need to tell their health care providers that they are taking it. The medications that St. John's wort interacts with are listed in **Table 11**.

St. John's Wort and Breastfeeding

St. John's wort is generally safe to take while breastfeeding (Dugoua et al., 2006; Hale, 2006; Humphrey, 2007). In a case study, Klier and colleagues

(2002) examined the pharmacokinetics of St. John's wort in four breastmilk samples (including both fore- and hindmilk) from a mother taking the standard dose of St. John's wort (300 mg/three times per day). They tested the samples for both hypericin and hyperforin and found that only hyperforin was excreted into breastmilk, at a low level. Both hyperforin and hypericin were below the level of quantification in the infant's plasma.

More recently, Klier and colleagues (2006) tested 36 breastmilk samples from five mothers taking 300 mg of St. John's wort, three times a day. They also tested the plasma of the five mothers and two infants. As with their earlier case study, they found that only hyperforin was excreted into breastmilk, at low levels. Hyperforin was at the limit of quantification in the infants' plasma, with the relative infant dose being 0.9% to 2.5% of the mother's dose. This level of infant exposure is comparable to that of antidepressants. No side effects were noted in either mothers or babies.

A recent review found that there is good evidence to support the use of St. John's wort while breastfeeding (Dugoua et al., 2006). The authors found that St. John's wort neither affects milk supply nor infant weight. They noted that it could cause infant colic, drowsiness, or lethargy, although only a few cases have been reported. The authors concluded that common and traditional use of St. John's wort caused minimal risk for breastfeeding women and their babies. They did express some concern about the use of St. John's wort during pregnancy, however.

Summary

St. John's wort is another effective alternative to antidepressants that may be more acceptable for some women. Its standard use is for mild-to-moderate depression, but it has also been used for major depression. Some cautions are in order. Even though St. John's wort is a "natural" alternative to medications, it is a medication and should be treated as such. It should never be used with antidepressants. Mothers need to tell their health care providers that they are taking it, as it can interact with a number of different medications. If used with safety concerns in mind, normal use of this medication does not appear to be harmful to mothers or babies. Although hyperforin is excreted into breastmilk, it appears in very low levels in infant plasma and in some cases was undetectable (Hale, 2006; Humphrey, 2007).

APPROACHES TO TREATMENT

All of the modalities described have been used by themselves to treat depression. Although mild-to-moderate depression is the standard indication for these modalities, most have also been successfully used for major depression. In addition, most of the modalities can be safely combined to increase their effectiveness. Indeed, combining modalities, such as exercise, EPA/DHA, and increased support, can create a synergistic effect. From a practical standpoint, be careful not to add too many options at once. Depressed mothers are likely to feel overwhelmed if there are too many things that they suddenly need to do. Combining two, possibly three, modalities may feel less overwhelming and more doable for depressed women.

If women are breastfeeding, their concerns about it need to be addressed up front. Some women will not seek treatment because they fear that they will be told to wean. Speaking from experience, that fear is realistic. Assure

Table 12: Combining Treatment Modalities		
Primary Treatment	**Other Treatments**	**Cautions**
Antidepressants	EPA/DHA Exercise Bright Light Therapy Social Support Psychotherapy	• Never combine St. John's wort with antidepressants. • In patients with bipolar disorder, limit morning light exposure and continue with medications during light treatment.
St. John's Wort	EPA/DHA Exercise Bright Light Therapy Social Support Psychotherapy	• Never combine with antidepressants. • St. John's wort may interact with other prescription medications.
EPA/DHA Exercise Bright Light Therapy Social Support Psychotherapy	Can all be combined with each other	• Be careful not to add so many modalities that mothers feel overwhelmed and have a hard time complying with treatment.

mothers that most treatments for depression are compatible with breastfeeding and that it is a priority to preserve breastfeeding whenever possible.

As described earlier, non-pharmacologic treatments can also be used as adjuncts to antidepressants. For example, bright light therapy, EPA/DHA, exercise, social support, and psychotherapy have been successfully used to boost the actions of medications when patients have had a partial response. St. John's wort is the only alternative treatment that can't be safely combined with antidepressants. **Table 12** summarizes safety issues for combining modalities.

For mothers who are reluctant to use antidepressants, a plan that includes non-pharmacologic treatments may persuade them to give medications a try. For example, they might talk with their health care providers about a trial of medications (e.g., 3 to 6 months), during which time, they could start exercising, increase their social support, and start taking EPA/DHA. After the trial period, mothers can be evaluated to see if they can taper off their medications. In the meantime, they have put other things in place to prevent a relapse. Many mothers are reluctant to take medications for fear that they will need to be on them "forever." With an end-point clearly in sight, they can address that fear in a concrete way and may be more open to a trial of medications.

An alternative scenario is for mothers to start with non-pharmacologic treatments, but monitor their progress. If they are not responding or are having a partial response after a discrete period (e.g., two months), evaluate the approach and consider adding or switching modalities. This can also be a time to revisit the issue of antidepressants. In any case, giving mothers options and finding out what they are willing to do will increase their compliance and facilitate their recovery.

CONCLUSIONS

Depression in new mothers needs to be treated promptly. For mothers who refuse antidepressants or for whom antidepressants may be inappropriate, we have more evidence-based options than ever before. These may prove more acceptable to patients, which mean that they may be more willing to seek treatment and comply once they begin. All of the choices described in this monograph are compatible with breastfeeding. This means that mothers are never forced to choose between their mental health and breastfeeding their babies—a choice no mother should have to make.

With the information in this monograph, health providers can help mothers make informed decisions on what they can do to alleviate their depression. For more information on postpartum depression, please see the resources listed in **Table 13.**

Table 13: For Further Information on Depression in New Mothers

Free curriculum on postpartum depression:
A Breastfeeding-Friendly Approach to Depression in New Mothers
This curriculum includes screening scales and current information on antidepressants and their compatibility with breastfeeding
www.NHBreastfeedingTaskForce.org

Resources for mothers: www.BreastfeedingMadeSimple.com

Resources for health care providers: www.GraniteScientific.com

---

REFERENCES

Abdel-Salam, O.M. (2005). Anti-inflammatory, antinociceptive, and gastric effects of Hypericum perforatum in rats. Scientific World Journal, 5, 586-595.

Akabas, S.R., & Deckelbaum, R.J. (2006). Summary of a workshop on n-3 fatty acids: Current status of recommendations and future directions. American Journal of Clinical Nutrition, 83, 1536-1538.

Amorin, A.R., Linne, Y.M., & Lourenco, P.M. (2007). Diet or exercise, or both, for weight reduction in women after childbirth. Cochrane Database Systematic Review, July 18.

Anghelescu, I.G., Kohnen, R., Szegedi, A., Klement, S., & Kieser, M. (2006). Comparison of Hypericum extract WS 5570 and paroxetine in ongoing treatment after recovery from an episode of moderate to severe depression: Results from a randomized multicenter study. Pharmacopsychiatry, 39, 213-219.

Antonuccio, D., Danton, W.G., & DeNelsky, G.Y. (1995). Psychotherapy versus medication for depression: Challenging the conventional wisdom with data. Professional Psychology: Research and Practice, 26, 574-585.

Appleby, L., Warner, R., Whitton, A., & Faragher, B. (1997). A controlled study of fluoxetine and cognitive-behavioral counseling in the treatment of postnatal depression. British Medical Journal, 314, 932-936.

Babyak, M., Blumenthal, J.A., Herman, S., Khatri, P., Doraiswamy, M., Moore, K., Craighead, W.E., Baldewicz, T.T., & Krishnan, R.R. (2000). Exercise treatment for major depression: Maintenance of therapeutic benefit at 10 months. Psychosomatic Medicine, 62, 633-638.

Balch, P. (2002). Prescription for herbal healing. New York: Avery.

Baxter, L.R., Schwartz, J.M., Bergman, K.S., & Szuba, M.P. (1992). Caudate glucose metabolic rate changes with both drug and behavioral therapy for obsessive-compulsive disorders. Archives of General Psychiatry, 49, 681-689.

Beck, C.T. (2001). Predictors of postpartum depression: An update. Nursing Research, 50, 275-285.

Blumenthal, J.A., Babyak, M.A., Doraiswamy, P.M., Watkins, L., Hoffman, B.M., Barbour, K.A., et al. (2007). Exercise and pharmacotherapy in the treatment of major depressive disorder. Psychosomatic Medicine, 69, 587-596.

Bradbury, J., Myers, S.P., & Oliver, C. (2005). An adaptogenic role for omega-3 fatty acids in stress: A randomized placebo controlled double blind intervention study. Nutrition Journal, 3(20), http://www.nutritionj.com/content/3/1/20.

Bratman, S., & Girman, A.M. (2003). Handbook of herbs and supplements and their therapeutic uses. St Louis: Mosby.

Brennan, P.A., Hammen, C., Anderson, M.J., Bor, W., Najman, J.M., & Williams, G.M. (2000). Chronicity, severity, and timing of maternal depressive symptoms: Relationships with child outcomes at age 5. Developmental Psychology, 36, 759-766.

Brummett, B.H., Siegler, I.C., Rohe, W.M., Barefoot, J.C., Vitaliano, P.P., Surwit, R.S., Feinglos, M.N., & Williams, R.B. (2005). Neighborhood characteristics moderate effects of caregiving on glucose functioning. Psychosomatic Medicine, 67, 752-758.

Carmichael, C.L., & Reis, H.T. (2005). Attachment, sleep quality, and depressed affect. Health Psychology, 24, 526-531.

Caughey, G. E., Mantzioris, E., Gibson, R. A., Cleland, L. G., & James, M. J. (1996). The effect on human tumor necrosis factor-alpha and interleukin 1-beta production of diets enriched in n-3 fatty acids from vegetable oil or fish oil. American Journal of Clinical Nutrition, 63, 116-122

Cheruku, S.R., Montgomery-Downs, H.E., Farkas, S.L., Thoman, E.B., & Lammi-Keefe, C.J. (2002). Higher maternal plasma docosahexaenoic acid during pregnancy is associated with more mature neonatal sleep-state patterning. American Journal of Clincial Nutrition, 76, 608-613.

Christensson, K., Siles, C., Moreno, L., Belaustequi, A., De La Fuente, P., Lagercrantz, H., et al. (1992). Temperature, metabolic adaptation and crying in healthy full-term newborns cared for skin-to-skin or in a cot. Acta Paediatr, 81(6-7), 488-493.

Cipriani, A., Geddes, J.R., Furukawa, T.A., & Barbui, C. (2007). Metareview on short-term effectiveness and safety of antidepressants for depression: An evidence-based approach to inform clinical practice. Canadian Journal of Psychiatry, 52, 553-562.

Cohen, S., Doyle, W.J., & Baum, A. (2006). Socioeconomic status is associated with stress hormones. Psychosomatic Medicine, 68, 414-420.

Cooper, P.J., Landman, M., Tomlinson, M., Molteno, C., Swartz, L., & Murray, L. (2002). Impact of a mother-infant intervention in an indigent peri-urban South African context: Pilot study. British Journal of Psychiatry, 180, 76-81.

Corral, M., Kuan, A., & Kostaras, D. (2000). Bright light therapy's effect on postpartum depression. American Journal of Psychiatry, 157, 303-304.

Corral, M., Wardrop, A.A., Zhang, H., Grewal, A.K., & Patton, S. (2007). Morning light therapy for postpartum depression. Archives of Women's Mental Health, 10, 221-224.

Coussons-Read, M.E., Okun, M.L., Schmitt, M.P., & Giese, S. (2005). Prenatal stress alters cytokine levels in a manner that may endanger human pregnancy. Psychosomatic Medicine, 67, 625-631.

Da Costa, D., Larouche, J., Dritsa, M., & Brender, W. (2000). Psychosocial correlates of prepartum and postpartum depressed mood. Journal of Affective Disorders, 59, 31-40.

Daley, A.J., Macarthur, C., & Winter, H. (2007). The role of exercise in treating postpartum depression: A review of the literature. Journal of Midwifery and Women's Health, 52, 56-62.

Dayan, J., Creveuil, C., Marks, M.N., Conroy, S., Herlicoviez, M., Dreyfus, M., & Tordjman, S. (2006). Prenatal depression, prenatal anxiety, and spontaneous preterm birth: A prospective cohort study among women with early and regular care. Psychosomatic Medicine, 68, 938-946.

Delarue, J., LeFoll, C., Corporeau, C., & Lucas, D. (2004). N-3 long-chain polyunsaturated fatty acids: A nutritional tool to prevent insulin resistance associated to type 2 diabetes and obesity? Reproductive Nutrition & Development, 44, 289-299.

Dell'Aica, I., Caniato, R., Biggin, S., & Garbisa, S. (2007). Matrix proteases, green tea, and St. John's wort: Biomedical research catches up with folk medicine. Clinical Chimica Acta, 381, 69-77.

Desan, P.H., Weinstein, A.J., Michalak, E.E., Tam, E.M., Meesters, Y., Ruiter, M.J., et al. (2007). A controlled trial of the Litebook light-emitting diode (LED) light therapy device for treatment of Seasonal Affective Disorder (SAD). BMC Psychiatry, 7, doi:10.1186/1471-1244X/1187/1138.

Dhabhar, F.D., & McEwen, B.S. (2001). Bidirectional effects of stress and glucocorticoid hormones on immune function: Possible explanations for paradoxical observations. In Ader R., Felten, D.L., & Cohen, N. (Ed.), Psychoneuroimmunology (Third Edition ed., Vol. 1 pp. 301-338). New York: Academic Press.

Dietz, P.M., Williams, S.B., Callaghan, W.M., Bachman, D.J., Whitlock, E.P., & Hornbrook, M.C. (2007). Clinically identified maternal depression before, during, and after pregnancies ending in live births. American Journal of Psychiatry, 164, 1515-1520.

Doering, L.V., Cross, R., Vredevoe, D., Martinez-Maza, O., & Cowan, M.J. (2007). Infection, depression and immunity in women after coronary artery bypass: A pilot study of cognitive behavioral therapy. Alternative Therapy, Health & Medicine, 13, 18-21.

Dugoua, J.J., Mills, E., Perri, D., & Koren, G. (2006). Safety and efficacy of St. John's wort (Hypericum) during pregnancy and lactation. Canadian Journal of Clinical Pharmacology, 13, e268-e276.

Dunstan, J.A., Roper, J., Mitoulas, L., Hartmann, P.E., Simmer, K., & Prescott, S.L. (2004). The effect of supplementation with fish oil during pregnancy on breast milk immunoglobulin A, soluble CD14, cytokine levels and fatty acid composition. Clinical & Experimental Allergy, 34, 1237-1242.

Dunstan, J.A., Mori, T.A., Barden, A., Beilin, L.J., Holt, P.G., Calder, P.C., Taylor, A.L., & Prescott, S.L. (2004). Effects of n-3 polyunsaturated fatty acid supplementation in pregnancy on maternal and fetal erythrocyte fatty acid composition. European Journal of Clinical Nutrition, 58, 429-437.

Eaker, E.D., Sullivan, L.M., Kelly-Hayes, M., D'Agostino, R.B., & Benjamin, E.J. (2007). Marital status, marital strain, and risk of coronary heart disease or total mortality: The Framingham Offspring Study. Psychosomatic Medicine, 69, 509-513.

Elliot, S.A., Leverton, T.J., Sanjack, M., Turner, H., Cowmeadow, P., Hopkins, J., & Bushnell, D. (2000). Promoting mental health after childbirth: A controlled trial of primary prevention of postnatal depression. British Journal of Clinical Psychology, 39, 223-241.

Emery, C.F., Kiecolt-Glaser, J.K., Glaser, R., Malarky, W.B., & Frid, D.J. (2005). Exercise accelerates wound healing among healthy older adults: A preliminary investigation. Journal of Gerontology, Series A, Biological Sciences and Medical Sciences, 60(11):1432-36.

Erman, M.K. (2007). Pharmacologic therapy: Melatonin, antidepressants, and other agents. Primary Psychiatry, 14, 21-24.

Ernst, E. (2002). The risk-benefit profile of commonly used herbal therapies: Ginkgo, St. John's wort, ginseng, echinacea, saw palmetto, and kava. Annals of Internal Medicine, 136, 42-53.

Evans, J., Heron, J., Francomb, H., Oke, S., & Golding, J. (2001). Cohort study of depressed mood during pregnancy and after childbirth. British Medical Journal, 323, 257-260.

Evans, J., Heron, J., Patel, R.R., & Wiles, N. (2007). Depressive symptoms during pregnancy and low birth weight at term. British Journal of Psychiatry, 191, 84-85.

Ferrucci, L., Cherubini, A., Bandinelli, S., Bartali, B., Corsi A., Lauretani, F., Martin, A., Andres-Lacueva, C., Senin, U., & Guralnik, J.M. (2006). Relationship of plasma polyunsaturated fatty acids to circulating inflammatory markers. Journal of Clinical Endocrinology & Metabolism, 91, 439-446.

Field, T., Diego, M., Hernandez-Reif, M., Schanberg, S., & Kuhn, C. (2002). Relative right versus left frontal EEG in neonates. Developmental Psychobiology, 41, 147-155.

Finucane, A., & Mercer, S.W. (2006). An exploratory mixed methods study of the acceptability and effectiveness of mindfulness-based cognitive therapy for patients with active depression and anxiety in primary care. BMC Psychiatry, 6(doi:10.11186/1471-244X-6-14).

Frangou, S., Lewis, M., & McCrone, P. (2006). Efficacy of ethyl-eicosapentaenoic acid in bipolar depression: Randomized double-blind placebo-controlled study. British Journal of Psychiatry, 188, 46-50.

Freeman, M.P., Hibbeln, J.R., Wisner, K.L., Davis, J.M., Mischoulon, D., Peet, M., Keck, P.E. Jr, , Marangell, L.B., Richardson, A.J., Lake, J., & Stoll, A.L. (2006a). Omega-3 fatty acids: Evidence basis for treatment and future research in psychiatry. Journal of Clinical Psychiatry, 67, 1954-1967.

Freeman, M.P. (2007). Antenatal depression: Navigating the treatment dilemmas. American Journal of Psychiatry, 164, 1162-1165.

Freeman, M.P., Hibbeln, J.R., H., Wisner, K.L., Brumbach, B.H., Watchman, M., & Gelenberg, A.J. (2006b). Randomized dose-ranging pilot trial of omega-3 fatty acids for postpartum depression. Acta Psychiatrica Scandanavica, 113, 31–35.

Gallo, L. C., Troxel, W.M., Matthews, K.A., & Kuller, L.H. (2003). Marital status and quality in middle-aged women: Associations with levels and trajectories of cardiovascular risk factors. Health Psychology, 22, 453-463.

Garland, M.R., Hallahan, B., McNamara, M., Carney, P.A., Grimes, H., Hibbeln, J.R., Harkin, A., & Conroy, R.M. (2007). Lipids and essential fatty acids in patients presenting with self-harm. British Journal of Psychiatry, 190, 112-117.

Geddes, J.R., Furukawa, T.A., Cipriani, A., & Barbui, C. (2007). Depressive disorder needs an evidence base commensurate with its public health importance. Canadian Journal of Psychiatry, 52, 543-544.

Goebel, M.U., Mills, P.J., Irwin, M.R., & Ziegler, M.G. (2000). Interleukin-6 and tumor necrosis factor-alpha production after acute psychological stress, exercise, and infused isoproterenol: Differential effects and pathways. Psychosomatic Research, 62, 591-598.

Golden, R.N., Gaynes, B.N., Ekstrom, R.D., Hamer, R.M., Jacobsen, F.M., Suppes, T., Wisner, K.L., & Nemeroff, C.B. (2005). The efficacy of light therapy in the treatment of mood disorders: A review and meta-analysis of the evidence. American Journal of Psychiatry, 162, 656-662.

Goodman, E., McEwen, B.S., Huang, B., Dolan, L.M., & Adler, N.E. (2005). Social inequalities in biomarkers of cardiovascular risk in adolescence. Psychosomatic Medicine, 67, 9-15.

Grandjean, P., Bjerve, K.S., Weihe, P., & Steuerwald, U. (2001). Birthweight in a fishing community: Significance of essential fatty acids and marine food contaminants. International Journal of Epidemiology, 30, 1272-1278.

Grigoriadis, S., & Ravitz, P. (2007). An approach to interpersonal psychotherapy for postpartum depression: Focusing on interpersonal changes. Canadian Family Physician, 53, 1469-1475.

Groër, M.W., Davis, M.W., Smith, K., Casey, K., Kramer, V., & Bukovsky, E. (2005). Immunity, inflammation and infection in post-partum breast and formula feeders. American Journal of Reproductive Immunology, 54, 222-231.

Groër, M.W., & Morgan, K. (2007). Immune, health and endocrine characteristics of depressed postpartum mothers. Psychoneuroendocrinology, 32(2), 133-139.

Hagan, R., Evans, S.F., & Pope, S. (2004). Preventing postnatal depression in mothers of very preterm infants: A randomized controlled trial. British Journal of Obstetrics & Gynecology, 111, 641-647.

Hale, T.W. (2006). Medications and mothers' milk (Vol. 12). Amarillo, TX: Hale Publishing.

Hallahan, B., & Garland, M.R. (2005). Essential fatty acids and mental health. British Journal of Psychiatry, 186, 275-277.

Hallahan, B., Hibbeln, J.R., Davis, J.M., & Garland, M.R. (2007). Omega-3 fatty acid supplementation in patients with recurrent self-harm. Single-centre double-blind randomized controlled trial. British Journal of Psychiatry, 190, 118-122.

Hamazaki, K., Itomura, M., Huan, M., Nishizawa, H., Sawazaki, S., Tanouchi, M. Watanabe, S., Hamazaki, T., Terasawa, K., & Yazawa, K. (2005). Effect of omega-3 fatty acid-containing phospholipids on blood catecholamine concentrations in healthy volunteers: A randomized, placebo-controlled, double-blind trial. Nutrition, 21, 705-710.

Hamer, M., & Steptoe, A. (2007). Association between physical fitness, parasympathetic control, and proinflammatory responses to mental stress. Psychosomatic Medicine, 69, 660-666.

Hammen, C., & Brennan, P. (2002). Interpersonal dysfunction in depressed women: Impairments independent of depressive symptoms. Journal of Affective Disorders, 72, 145-156.

Harkness, R., & Bratman, S. (2003). Handbook of drug-herb and drug-supplement interactions. St. Louis, MO: Mosby.

Haslam, D.M., Pakenham, K.I., & Smith, A. (2006). Social support and postpartum depressive symptomatogy: The mediating role of maternal self-efficacy. Infant Mental Health Journal, 27, 276-291.

Hassmen, P., Koivula, N., & Uutela, A. (2000). Physical exercise and psychological well-being: A population study in Finland. Preventative Medicine, 30, 17-25.

Hawkes, J.S., Bryan, D.L., Makrides, M., Neumann, M.A., & Gibson, R.A. (2002). A randomized trial of supplementation with docosahexaenoic acid-rich tuna oil and its effects on the human milk cytokines interleukin 1-β, interleukin 6, and tumor necrosis factor α. American Journal of Clinical Nutrition, 75, 754-760.

Hayes, B.A., Muller, R., & Bradley, B.S. (2001). Perinatal depression: A randomized controlled trial of an antenatal education intervention for primiparas. Birth, 28, 28-35.

Helland, I.B., Smith, L., Saarem, K., Saugstad, O.D., & Drevon, C.A. (2003). Maternal supplementation with very-long-chain n-3 fatty acids during pregnancy and lactation augments children's IQ at 4 years of age. Pediatrics, 111, e39-e44.

Hendrick, V. (2003). Treatment of postnatal depression. British Medical Journal, 327, 1003-1004.

Hibbeln, J.R. (2002). Seafood consumption, the DHA content of mothers' milk and prevalence rates of postpartum depression: A cross-national, ecological analysis. Journal of Affective Disorders, 69, 15-29.

Hobfoll, S.E., Ritter, C., Lavin, J., Hulsizer, M.R., & Cameron, R.P. (1995). Depression prevalence and incidence among inner-city pregnant and postpartum women. Journal of Consulting and Clinical Psychology, 63, 445-453.

Hong, S., Nelesen, R.A., Krohn, P.L., Mills, P.J., & Dimsdale, J.E. (2006). The association of social status and blood pressure with markers of vascular inflammation. Psychosomatic Medicine, 68, 517-523.

Hu, Z.P., Yang, X.X., Chan, S.Y., Xu A.L., Duan, W., Zhu, Y.Z., et al. (2006). St. John's wort attenuates irinotecan-induced diarrhea via down-regulation of intestinal pro-inflammatory cytokines and inhibition of intestinal epithelial apoptosis. Toxicology & Applied Pharmacology, 216, 225-237.

Humphrey, S. (2003). The nursing mother's herbal. Minneapolis: Fairview Press.

Humphrey, S. (2007). Herbal therapeutics during lactation. In Hale, T.W. & Hartmann, P.E. (Eds.), Textbook of Human Lactation (pp. 629-654). Amarillo, TX: Hale Publishing.

Hypericum Depression Trial Study Group. (2002). Effect of Hypericum perforatum (St. John's Wort) in major depressive disorder. Journal of the American Medical Association, 287, 1807-1814.

Institute for Natural Products Research (2000). Pocket Reference Guide to Botanical and Dietary Supplements. Marine on St. Croix, MN: Institute for Natural Products Research.

Jensen, C.L. (2006). Effects of n-3 fatty acids during pregnancy and lactation. American Journal of Clinical Nutrition, 83, 1452S-1457S.

Jones, N.A., McFall, B.A., & Diego, M.A. (2004). Patterns of brain electrical activity in infants of depressed mothers who breastfeed and bottle feed: The mediating role of infant temperament. Biological Psychology, 67, 103-124.

Kendall-Tackett, K.A. (2005). Depression in new mothers: Causes, consequences and treatment options. Binghamton, New York: Haworth Press.

Kendall-Tackett, K.A. (2007b). Cardiovascular disease and metabolic syndrome as sequelae of violence against women: A psychoneuroimmunology approach. Trauma, Violence and Abuse, 8, 117-126.

Kendall-Tackett, K.A. (2007a). A new paradigm for depression in new mothers: The central role of inflammation and how breastfeeding and anti-inflammatory treatments protect maternal mental health. International Breastfeeding Journal, 2:6(http://www.internationalbreastfeedingjournal.com/content/2/1/6).

Kew, S., Banerjee, T., Minihane, A.M., Finnegan, Y.E., Muggli, R., Albers, R., et al. (2003). Lack of effect of foods enriched with plant- or marine-derived n-3 fatty acids on human immune function. American Journal of Clinical Nutrition, 77, 1287-1295.

Kew, S., Mesa, M.D., Tricon, S., Buckley, R., Minihane, A.M., & Yaqoob, P. (2004). Effects of oils rich in eicosapentaenoic and docosahexanoic acids on immune cell composition and function in healthy humans. American Journal of Clinical Nutrition, 79, 674-681.

Kiecolt-Glaser, J. K., & Newton, T.L. (2001). Marriage and health: His and hers. Psychological Bulletin, 127, 472-503.

Kiecolt-Glaser, J.K., Loving, T.J., Stowell, J.R., Malarky, W.B., Lemeshow, S., Dickinson, S.L., & Glaser, R. (2005). Hostile marital interactions, proinflammatory cytokine production, and wound healing. Archives of General Psychiatry, 62, 1377-1384.

Kiecolt-Glaser, J.K., Belury, M.A., Porter, K., Beversdoft, D., Lemeshow, S., & Glaser, R. (2007). Depressive symptoms, omega-6: omega-3 fatty acids, and inflammation in older adults. Psychosomatic Medicine, 69, 217-224.

Klier, C.M., Muzik, M., Rosenblum, K.L., & Lenz, G. (2001). Interpersonal psychotherapy adapted for the group setting in the treatment of postpartum depression. Journal of Psychotherapy Practice and Research, 10, 124-131.

Klier, C.M., Schafer, M.R., Schmid-Siegel, B., Lenz, G., & Mannel, M. (2002). St. John's wort (Hypericum Perforatum)—Is it safe during breastfeeding? Pharmacopsychiatry, 35, 29-30.

Klier, C.M., Schmid-Siegel, B., Schafer, M.R., Lenz, G., Saria, A., Lee, A., & Zernig, G. (2006). St. John's wort (Hypericum perforatum) and breastfeeding: Plasma and breast milk concentrations of hyperforin for 5 mothers and 2 infants. Journal of Clinical Psychiatry, 67, 305-309.

Kohut, M.L., McCann, D.A., Konopka, D.W.R., Cunnick, J.E., Franke, W.D., Castillo, M.C., & Vanderah, R.E. (2006). Aerobic exercise, but not flexibility/resistance exercise, reduces serum IL-18, CRP, and IL-6 independent of β-blockers, BMI, and psychosocial factors in older adults. Brain, Behavior, & Immunity, 20, 201-209.

Konsman, J.P., Parnet, P., & Dantzer, R. (2002). Cytokine-induced sickness behaviour: Mechanisms and implications. Trends in Neuroscience, 25, 154-158.

Kop, W.J., Berman, D.S., Gransar, H., Wong, N.D., Miranda-Peats, R., White, M.D., et al. (2005). Social networks and coronary artery calcification in asymptomatic individuals. Psychosomatic Medicine, 67, 343-352.

Kop, W.J., & Gottdiener, J.S. (2005). The role of immune system parameters in the relationship between depression and coronary artery disease. Psychosomatic Medicine, 67, S37-S41.

Kuhn, M.A., & Winston, D. (2000). Herbal therapy and supplements: A scientific and traditional approach. Philadelphia, PA: Lippincott.

Lam, R.W., Song, C., & Yatham, L.N. (2004). Does neuroimmune dysfunction mediate seasonal mood changes in winter depression? Medical Hypotheses, 63, 567-573.

Lam, R.W., Levitt, A.J., Levitan, R.D., Enns, M.W., Morehouse, R., Michalak, E.E., & Tam, E.M. (2006). The CAN-SAD Study: A randomized controlled trial of the effectiveness of light therapy and fluoxetine in patients with winter seasonal affective disorder. American Journal of Psychiatry, 163, 805-812.

Lane, A.M., Crone-Grant, D., & Lane, H. (2002). Mood changes following exercise. Perceptual & Motor Skills, 94, 732-734.

Lawvere, S., & Mahoney, M.C. (2005). St. John's wort. American Family Physician, 72, 2249-2254.

Lecrubier, Y., Clerc, G., Didi, R., & Kieser, M. (2002). Efficacy of St. John's wort extract WS 5570 in major depression: A double-blind, placebo-controlled trial. American Journal of Psychiatry, 159, 1361-1366.

Letourneau, N., Duffett-Leger, L., Stewart, M., Hegadoren, K., Dennis, C.L., Rinaldi, C. M., et al. (2007). Canadian mothers' perceived support needs during postpartum depression. Journal of Obstetric, Gynecologic, and Neonatal Nursing, 36, 441-449.

Leu, S.J., Shiah, I.S., Yatham, L.N., Cheu, Y.M., & Lam, R.W. (2001). Immune-inflammatory markers in patients with seasonal affective disorder: Effects of light therapy. Journal of Affective Disorders, 63, 27-34.

Lewis, T., Amini, F., & Lannon, R. (2000). A general theory of love. New York: Vintage.

Lewis, T.T., Everson-Rose, S.A., Powell, L.H., Matthews, K.A., Brown, C., Karavolos, K., et al. (2006). Chronic exposure to everyday discrimination and coronary artery calcification in African American women: The SWAN Heart Study. Psychosomatic Medicine, 68, 362-368.

Linde, K., Ramirez, G., Mulrow, C.D., Pauls, A., Weidenhammer, W., & Melchart, D. (1996). St. John's wort for depression: An overview and meta-analysis of randomized clinical trials. British Medical Journal, 313, 253-258.

Llorente, A.M., Jensen, C.L., Voigt, R.G., Fraley, J.K., Berretta, M.C., & Heird, W.C. (2003). Effect of maternal docosahexaenoic acid supplementation on postpartum depression and information processing. American Journal of Obstetrics & Gynecology, 188, 1348-1353.

LoCicero, A.K., Weiss, D.M., & Issokson, D. (1997). Postpartum depression: Proposal for prevention through an integrated care and support network. Applied and Preventive Psychology, 6, 169-178.

Looper, K.J. (2007). Potential medical and surgical complications of sertonergic antidepressant medications. Psychosomatics, 48, 1-9.

Loucks, E.B., Berkman, L.F., Cruenewald, T.L., & Seeman, T.E. (2005). Social integration is associated with fibrinogen concentration in elderly men. Psychosomatic Medicine, 67, 353-358.

Louik, C., Lin, A.E., Werler, M.M., Hernandez-Diaz, S., & Mitchell, A.A. (2007). First-trimester use of selective serotonin-reuptake inhibitors and the risk of birth defects. New England Journal of Medicine, 356, 2675-2683.

Lowe, N.K. (2007). Highlights of The Listening to Mothers II Survey. Journal of Obstetric, Gynecologic and Neonatal Nursing, 36, 1-2.

Luoma, I., Tamminen, T., Kaukonen, P., Laippala, P., Puura, K., Salelin, R., & Almqvist, F. (2001). Longitudinal study of maternal depressive symptoms and child well-being. Journal of the American Academy of Child and Adolescent Psychiatry, 40, 1367-1374.

MacArthur, C., Winter, H.R., Bick, D.E., Knowles, H., Lilford, R., Henderson, C., Lancashire, R.J., Braunholtz, D.A., & Gee, H. (2002). Effects of redesigned community postnatal care on women's health 4 months after birth: A cluster randomized controlled trial. Lancet, 359, 378-385.

Maes, M., & Smith, R.S. (1998). Fatty acids, cytokines, and major depression. Biological Psychiatry, 43, 313-314.

Maes, M. (2001). Psychological stress and the inflammatory response system. Clinical Science, 101, 193-194.

Maes, M., Christophe, A., Bosmans, E., Lin, A., & Neels, H. (2000). In humans, serum polyunsaturated fatty acid levels predict the response of proinflammatory cytokines to psychologic stress. Biological Psychiatry, 47, 910-920.

Malcolm, C.A., McCulloch, D.L., Montgomery, C., Shepherd, A., & Weaver, L.T. (2003). Maternal docosahexaenoic acid supplementation during pregnancy and visual evoked potential development in term infants: A double-blind, prospective, randomized trial. Archives of Diseases of Childhood, Fetal, and Neonatal Education, 88, 383-390.

Marangell, L.B., Martinez, J.M., Zboyan, H.A., Chong, H., & Puryear, L.J. (2004). Omega-3 fatty acids for the prevention of postpartum depression: Negative data from a preliminary, open-label pilot study. Depression & Anxiety, 19, 20-23.

Mather, A.S., Rodriguez, C., Guthrie, M.F., McHarg, A.M., Reid, I.C., & McMurdo, M.E.T. (2002). Effects of exercise on depressive symptoms in older adults with poorly responsive depressive disorder: Randomized controlled trial. British Journal of Psychiatry, 180, 411-415.

McAuley, E., Blissmer, B., Katula, J., Duncan, T.E., & Mihalko, S.L. (2000). Physical activity, self-esteem, and self-efficacy relationships in older adults:

A randomized controlled trial. Annals of Behavioral Medicine, 22, 131-139.

McDade, T.W., Hawkley, L.C., & Cacioppo, J.T. (2006). Psychosocial and behavioral predictors of inflammation in middle-aged and older adults: The Chicago Health, Aging, and Social Relations Study. Psychosomatic Medicine, 68, 376-381.

McEwen, B. S. (2003). Mood disorders and allostatic load. Biological Psychiatry, 54, 200-207.

Milgrom, J., Negri, L.M., Gemmill, A.W., McNeil, M., & Martin, P.R. (2005). A randomized controlled trial of psychological interventions for postnatal depression. British Journal of Clinical Psychology, 44, 529-542.

Miller, G.E., Cohen, S., & Ritchey, A.K. (2002). Chronic psychological stress and the regulation of pro-inflammatory cytokines: A glucocorticoid-resistance model. Health Psychology, 21, 531-541.

Miller, G.E., Rohleder, N., Stetler, C., & Kirschbaum, C. (2005). Clinical depression and regulation of the inflammatory response during acute stress. Psychosomatic Medicine, 67, 679-687.

Misri, S., Reebye, P., Corral, M., & Mills, L. (2004). The use of paroxetine and cognitive-behavioral therapy in postpartum depression and anxiety: A randomized controlled trial. Journal of Clinical Psychiatry, 65, 1236-1241.

Miyake, Y., Sasaki, S., Yokoyama, T., Tanaka, K., Ohya, Y., Fukushima, W., et al. (2006). Risk of postpartum depression in relation to dietary fish and fat intake in Japan: The Osaka Maternal and Child Health Study. Psychological Medicine, 36, 1727-1735.

Mohrbacher, N., & Kendall-Tackett, K.A. (2005). Breastfeeding made simple: Seven natural laws for nursing mothers. Oakland, CA: New Harbinger.

Morrell, C.J., Spiby, H., Stewart, P., Walters, S., & Morgan, A. (2000). Costs and effectiveness of community postnatal support workers: Randomised controlled trial. British Medical Journal, 321, 593-598.

Mufson, L., Dorta, K.P., Wickramaratne, P., Nomura, Y., Olfson, M., & Weissman, M.M. (2004). A randomized effectiveness trial of interpersonal psychotherapy for depressed adolescents. Archives of General Psychiatry, 61, 577-584.

Muller, W.E. (2003). Current St. John's wort research from mode of action to clinical efficacy. Pharmacology Research, 47, 101-109.

National Alliance on Mental Illness (NAMI). (2007). Seasonal affective disorder. www.nami.org.

Nemets, B., Stahl, Z., & Belmaker, R.H. (2002). Addition of omega-3 fatty acid to maintenance medication treatment for recurrent unipolar depressive disorder. American Journal of Psychiatry, 159, 477-479.

Nemets, H., Nemets, B., Apter, A., Bracha, Z., & Belmaker, R.H. (2006). Omega-3 treatment of childhood depression: A controlled, double-blind pilot study. American Journal of Psychiatry, 163, 1098-1100.

Noaghiul, S., & Hibbeln, J.R. (2003). Cross-national comparisons of seafood consumption and rates of bipolar disorders. American Journal of Psychiatry, 160, 2222-2227.

O'Hara, M.W., Stuart, S., Gorman, L.L., & Wenzel, A. (2000). Efficacy of interpersonal psychotherapy for postpartum depression. Archives of General Psychiatry, 57, 1039-1045.

O'Hara, M.W., & Swain, A.M. (1996). Rates and risk of postpartum depression: A meta-analysis. International Review of Psychiatry, 8, 37-54.

Olafsdottir, A.S., Skuladottir, G.V., Thorsdottir, I., Hauksson, A., Thorgeirsdottir, H., & Steingrimsdottir, L. (2006). Relationship between high consumption of marine fatty acids in early pregnancy and hypertensive disorders in pregnancy. British Journal of Obstetrics & Gynecology, 113, 301-309.

Olfson, M., Marcus, S.C., Tedeschi, M., & Wan, G.J. (2006). Continuity of antidepressant treatment for adults with depression in the United States. American Journal of Psychiatry, 163, 101-108.

Olsen, S.F., Secher, N.J., Tabor, A., Weber, T., Walker, J.J., & Gluud, C. (2000). Randomised clinical trials of fish oil supplementation in high-risk populations. British Journal of Obstetrics & Gynaecology, 107, 382-395.

Oren, D.A., Wisner, K.L., Spinelli, M., Epperson, C.N., Peindl, K.S., Terman, J.S., & Terman, M. (2002). An open trial of morning light therapy for treatment of antepartum depression. American Journal of Psychiatry, 159, 666-669.

Orr, S.T., Reiter, J.P., Blazer, D.G., & James, S.A. (2007). Maternal prenatal pregnancy-related anxiety and spontaneous preterm birth in Baltimore, Maryland. Psychosomatic Medicine, 69, 566-570.

Orth-Gomer, K., Wamala, S.P., Horsten, M., Schenk-Gustafsson, K., Schneiderman, N., & Mittleman, M.A. (2000). Marital stress worsens prognosis in women with coronary heart disease: The Stockholm Female Coronary Risk Study. Journal of the American Medical Association, 284, 3008-3014.

Parker, G., Gibson, N.A., Brotchie, H., Heruc, G., Rees, A.M., & Hadzi-Pavlovic, D. (2006). Omega-3 fatty acids and mood disorders. American Journal of Psychiatry, 163, 969-978.

Patel, V., Rodrigues, M., & DeSouza, N. (2002). Gender, poverty, and postnatal depression: A study of mothers in Goa, India. American Journal of Psychiatry, 159, 43-47.

Patel, V., & Prince, M. (2006). Maternal psychological morbidity and low birth weight in India. British Journal of Psychiatry, 188, 284-285.

Payne, J.L. (2007). Antidepressant use in the postpartum period: Practical considerations. American Journal of Psychiatry, 164, 1329-1332.

Peet, M., & Horrobin, D.F. (2002). A dose-ranging study of the effects of ethyl-eicosapentaenoate in patients with ongoing depression despite apparently adequate treatment with standard drugs. Archives General Psychiatry, 59, 913-919.

Peet, M., & Stokes, C. (2005). Omega-3 fatty acids in the treatment of psychiatric disorders. Drugs, 65, 1051-1059.

Philipp, M., Kohnen, R., & Hiller, K.O. (1999). Hypericum extract versus imipramine or placebo in patients with moderate depression: Randomized multicenter study of treatment for eight weeks. British Medical Journal, 319, 1534-1539.

Prasko, J., Horocek, J., Zalesky, R., Kopecek, M., Novak, T., Paskova, B., et al. (2004). The change of regional brain metabolism (18FDG PET) in panic disorder during the treatment with cognitive behavioral therapy or antidepressants. Neuro Endocrinology Letters, 25, 340-348.

Quinn, T.J., & Carey, G.B. (1999). Does exercise intensity or diet influence lactic acid accumulation in breast milk? Medicine and Science in Sports and Exercise, 31, 105-110.

Ranjit, N., Diez-Roux, A.V., Shea, S., Cushman, M., Seeman, T., Jackson, S.A., & Ni, H. (2007). Psychosocial factors and inflammation in the Multi-Ethnic Study of Atherosclerosis. Archives of Internal Medicine, 167, 174-181.

Reay, R., Fisher, Y., Robertson, M., Adams, E., Owen, C., & Kumar, R. (2006). Group interpersonal psychotherapy for postnatal depression: A pilot study. Archives of Women's Mental Health, 9, 31-39.

Rees, A.M., Austin, M.P., & Parker, G. (2005). Role of omega-3 fatty acids as a treatment for depression in the perinatal period. Australia & New Zealand Journal of Psychiatry, 39, 274-280.

Rich, M., Currie, J., & McMahon, C. (2004). Physical exercise and the lactating woman: A qualitative pilot study of mothers' perceptions and experiences. Breastfeeding Review, 12, 11-17.

Ritter, C., Hobfoll, S.E., Lavin, J., Cameron, R.P., & Hulsizer, M.R. (2000). Stress, psychosocial resources, and depressive symptomatology during pregnancy in low-income, inner-city women. Health Psychology, 19, 576-585.

Robles, T.F., Glaser, R., & Kiecolt-Glaser, J.K. (2005). Out of balance: A new look at chronic stress, depression, and immunity. Current Directions in Psychological Science, 14, 111-115.

Roux, G., Anderson, C., & Roan, C. (2002). Postpartum depression, marital dysfunction, and infant outcome: A longitudinal study. Journal of Perinatal Education, 11, 25-36.

Rupke, S.J., Blecke, D., & Renfrow, M. (2006). Cognitive therapy for depression. American Family Physician, 73, 83-86.

Sarris, J. (2007). Herbal medicines in the treatment of psychiatric disorders: A systematic review. Phytotherapy Research, 21, 703-716.

Schultz, V. (2006). Safety of St. John's wort extract compared to synthetic antidepressants. Phytomedicine, 13, 199-204.

Seng, J.S., Oakley, D.J., Sampselle, C.M., Killion, C., Graham-Bermann, S., & Liberzon, I. (2001). Posttraumatic stress disorder and pregnancy complications. Obstetrics & Gynecology, 97, 17-22.

Shoji, H., Franke, C., Campoy, C., Rivero, M., Demmelmair, H., & Koletzko, B. (2006). Effect of docosahexaenoic acid and eicosapentaenoic acid supplementation on oxidative stress levels during pregnancy. Free Radical Research, 40, 379-384.

Simon, G.E., VonKorff, M., Rutter, C., & Wagner, E. (2000). Randomised trial of monitoring, feedback, and management of care by telephone to improve treatment of depression in primary care. British Medical Journal, 320, 550-554.

Singh, N.A., Clements, K.M., & Fiatarone Singh, M.A. (2001). The efficacy of exercise as a long-term antidepressant in elderly subjects: A randomized, controlled trial. Journal of Gerontology, 56A, M497-M504.

Smuts C.M., Huang, M., Mundy, D., Plasse, T., Major, S., & Carlson, S.E. (2003). A randomized trial of docosahexaenoic acid supplementation during the third trimester of pregnancy. Obstetrics & Gynecology, 101, 469-479.

Spinelli, M.G., & Endicott, J. (2003). Controlled clinical trial of interpersonal psychotherapy versus parenting education program for depressed pregnant women. American Journal of Psychiatry, 160, 555-562.

Starkweather, A.R. (2007). The effects of exercise on perceived stress and IL-6 levels among older adults. Biological Nursing Research, 8, 1-9.

Stuart, S., & O'Hara, M.W. (1995). Interpersonal psychotherapy for postpartum depression. Journal of Psychotherapy Practice and Research, 4, 18-29.

Su, D., Zhao, Y., Binna, C., Scott, J., & Oddy, W. (2007). Breast-feeding mothers can exercise: Results of a cohort study. Public Health Nutrition, 10, 1089-1093.

Suarez, E.C., Lewis, J.G., Krishnan, R.R., & Young, K.H. (2004). Enhanced expression of cytokines and chemokines by blood monocytes to in vitro lipopolysaccharide stimulation are associated with hostility and severity of depressive symptoms in healthy women. Psychoneuroendocrinology, 29, 1119-1128.

Suarez, E.C. (2006). Sex differences in the relation of depressive symptoms, hostility, and anger expression to indices of glucose metabolism in nondiabetic adults. Health Psychology, 25, 484-492.

Sublette, M.E., Hibbeln, J.R., Galfalvy, H., Oquendo, M.A., & Mann, J.J. (2006). Omega-3 polyunsaturated essential fatty acid status as a predictor of future suicide risk. American Journal of Psychiatry, 163, 1100-1102.

Sullivan, B., & Payne, T.W. (2007). Affective disorders and cognitive failures: A comparison of seasonal and nonseasonal depression. American Journal of Psychiatry, 164, 1663-1667.

Suri, R., Altshuler, L., Hellemann, G., Burt, V.K., Aquino, A., & Mintz, J. (2007). Effects of antenatal depression and antidepressant treatment on gestational age at birth and risk of preterm birth. American Journal of Psychiatry, 164, 1206-1213.

Szegedi, A., Kohnen, R., Dienel, A., & Kieser, M. (2005). Acute treatment of moderate to severe depression with hypericum extract WS 5570 (St. John's wort): Randomised controlled double blind non-inferiority trial versus paroxetine. British Medical Journal, 330, 503.

Tanskanen, A., Hibbeln, J.R., Tuomilehto, J., Uutela, A., Haukkala, A., Viinamaki, H., Lehtonen, J., & Vartiainen, E. (2001). Fish consumption and depressive symptoms in the general population of Finland. Psychiatric Service, 52, 529-531.

Terman, M., & Terman, J.S. (2005). Light therapy for seasonal and nonseasonal depression: Efficacy, protocol, safety, and side effects. CNS Spectrums, 10, 647-663.

Terman, M., & Terman, J.S. (2006). Controlled trial of naturalistic dawn simulation and negative air ionization for Seasonal Affective Disorder. American Journal of Psychiatry, 163, 2126.

Tolman, A.O. (2001). Depression in adults: The latest assessment and treatment strategies. Kansas City, MO: Compact Clinicals.

Troxel, W.M., Cyranowski, J.M., Hall, M., Frank, E., & Buysee, D.J. (2007). Attachment anxiety, relationship context, and sleep in women with recurrent major depression. Psychosomatic Medicine, 69, 692-699.

Van Gurp, G., Meterissian, G.B., Haiek, L.N., McCusker, J., & Bellavance, F. (2002). St. John's wort or sertraline? Randomized controlled trial in primary care. Canadian Family Physician, 48, 905-912.

Wang, C., Chung, M., Lichtenstein, A., Balk, E., Kupelnick, B., DeVine, D., et al. (2004). Effects of omega-3 fatty acids on cardiovascular disease (Vol. AHRQ Publication No. 04-E009-1). Rockville, MD: Agency for Healthcare Research and Quality.

Webster, J., Linnane, J.W.J., Dibley, L.M., Hinson, J.K., Starrenburg, S.E., & Roberts, J.A. (2000a). Measuring social support in pregnancy: Can it be simple and meaningful? Birth, 27, 97-101.

Webster, J., Linnane, J.W.J., Dibley, L.M., & Pritchard, M. (2000b). Improving antenatal recognition of women at risk for postnatal depression. Australia and New Zealand Journal of Obstetrics and Gynaecology, 40, 409-412.

Weinberg, M.K., Tronick, E.Z., Beeghly, M., Olson, K.L., Kernan, H., & Riley, J.M. (2001). Subsyndromal depressive symptoms and major depression in postpartum women. American Journal of Orthopsychiatry, 71, 87-97.

Weisse, C.S. (1992). Depression and immunocompetence: A review of the literature. Psychological Bulletin, 111, 475-489.

Weissman, M.M., Wickramaratne, P., Nomura, Y., Warner, V., Pilowsky, D., & Verdeli, H. (2006). Offspring of depressed parents: 20 years later. American Journal of Psychiatry, 163, 1001-1008.

Weissman, M.M. (2007). Recent non-medication trials of interpersonal psychotherapy for depression. International Journal of Neuropsychopharmacology, 10, 117-122.

Werneke, U., Turner, T., & Priebe, S. (2006). Complementary medicines in psychiatry: Review of effectiveness and safety. British Journal of Psychiatry, 188, 109-121.

Whiskey, E., Werneke, U., & Taylor, D. (2001). A systematic review and meta-analysis of Hypericum perforatum in depression: A comprehensive clinical review. International Clinical Psychopharmacology, 16, 239-252.

Wilson, C.J., Finch, C.E., & Cohen, H.J. (2002). Cytokines and cognition—The case for a head-to-toe inflammatory paradigm. Journal of the American Geriatrics Society, 50, 2041-2056.

Woelk, H. (2000). Comparison of St. John's wort and imipramine for treating depression: Randomised controlled trial. British Medical Journal, 321, 536-539.

Wurglies, M., & Schubert-Zsilavecz, M. (2006). Hypericum perforatum: A "modern" herbal antidepressant: Pharmacokinetics of active ingredients. Clinical Pharmacokinetics, 45, 449-468.

Yonkers, K.A., Ramin, S.M., Rush, A.J., Navarrete, C.A., Carmody, T., March, D., Heartwell, S.F., & Leveno, K.J. (2001). Onset and persistence of postpartum depression in an inner-city maternal health clinic system. American Journal of Psychiatry, 158, 1856-1863.

Yonkers, K.A. (2007). The treatment of women suffering from depression who are either pregnant or breastfeeding. American Journal of Psychiatry, 164, 1457-1459.

Zanardo, V., Golin, R., Amato, M., Trevisanuto, D., Favaro, F., Faggian, D., & Plebani, M. (2007). Cytokines in human colostrum and neonatal jaundice. Pediatric Research, 62, 191-194.

Zanarini, M.C., & Frankenburg, F.R. (2003). Omega-3 fatty acid treatment of women with Borderline Personality Disorder: A double-blind, placebo-controlled pilot study. American Journal of Psychiatry, 160, 167-169.

Zanoli, P. (2004). Role of hyperforin in the pharmacological activities of St. John's wort. CNS, 10, 203-218.

Zhou, C., Tabb, M.M., Sadatrafiei, A., Grun, F., Sun, A., & Blumberg, B. (2004). Hyperforin, the active component of St. John's wort, induces IL-8 expression in human intestinal epithelial cells via a MAPK-dependent, NF-kappaB-independent pathway. Journal of Clinical Immunology, 24, 623-636.

Zlotnick, C., Miller, I.W., Pearlstein, T., Howard, M., & Sweeney, P. (2006). A preventive intervention for pregnant women on public assistance at risk for postpartum depression. American Journal of Psychiatry, 163, 1443-1445.

GLOSSARY

AA: arachidonic acid

ACTH: adrenocorticotropin hormone

ALA: alpha-linolenic acid

CRH: corticotrophin releasing hormone

CRP: C-reactive protein

DHA: docosahexanoic acid

EEG: electroencephalogram

EPA: eicosapentenoic acid

ET-1: endothelin-1

GLA: gamma-linoleic acid

HPA-axis: hypothalamic pituitary adrenal axis

ICAM: intercellular adhesion molecule

IFN-γ: interferon-γ

IL-1α: interleukin-1α

IL-1β: interleukin-1β

IL-6: interleukin-6

IL-8: interleukin-8

IL-10: interleukin-10

LA: linoleic acid

PUFA: polyunsaturated fatty acids

SAD: seasonal affective disorder

sICAM: soluble intercellular adhesion molecule

SSRIs: Selective serotonin reuptake inhibitors

TNF-α: tumor necrosis factor-α

USP: U.S. Pharmacoepia

UV: ultraviolet

INDEX

AUTHOR BIOGRAPHY

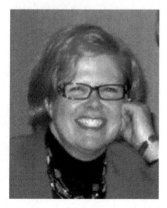

Kathleen Kendall-Tackett, Ph.D., IBCLC, is a health psychologist and International Board Certified Lactation Consultant, specializing in women's health. She is a Research Associate at the Family Research Lab, an Affiliate Research Associate Professor of Psychology at the University of New Hampshire, and a Fellow of the American Psychological Association in both the Divisions of Health Psychology and Trauma Psychology. Dr. Kendall-Tackett is a La Leche League Leader, chair of the New Hampshire Breastfeeding Taskforce, and the Area Coordinator of Leaders for La Leche League of Maine and New Hampshire.

92328178R00055

Made in the USA
Lexington, KY
02 July 2018